Looking like

You

A Word From Joel Clark Kira

When I met Barry Hendrickson in the mid 80's in N.Y. he had done everything imaginable in wig design. Fantasy Mohawks gave way to stunningly natural looks as he evolved into his own salon.

By happenstance, many clients began to recommend him to family members who were going through chemotherapy. From asking about their experience, and learning about their concerns and needs, he realized "we need to work on the inside of the head before we work on the outside."

During the consultation he outlines step by step what to expect during the treatments, showing exciting options for hair replacement. He consistently achieves amazing results not only for their looks, but also more significantly for their outlook.

An influential journalist was stunned at the boost to her friend's morale in just one visit. In the New York Times she proclaimed, "Hendrickson and company are nothing short of guardian angels."

It became obvious that an illustrated guidebook would make things easier for everyone. Many moons of our writing experimentation and perfecting have resulted in "Looking Like You."

It has been rewarding to observe this journey and collaborate capturing the spirit and practical wisdom for everyone.

Putting it together bit-by-bit, piece-by-piece.

We found Soraya Spahi straight out of a prestigious school of design, where her spectacular portfolio won top honors in her graduating class. Her refreshing style resonated with Barry's vision. Like the artist herself, every page sparkles with inspiration.

It has honestly been the thrill of a lifetime for all of us to bring such a worthy project to life. As a team, we are excited to see the continued success for anyone who needs and reads . . . "Looking Like You."

. . . . *Joel*

Table of Contents

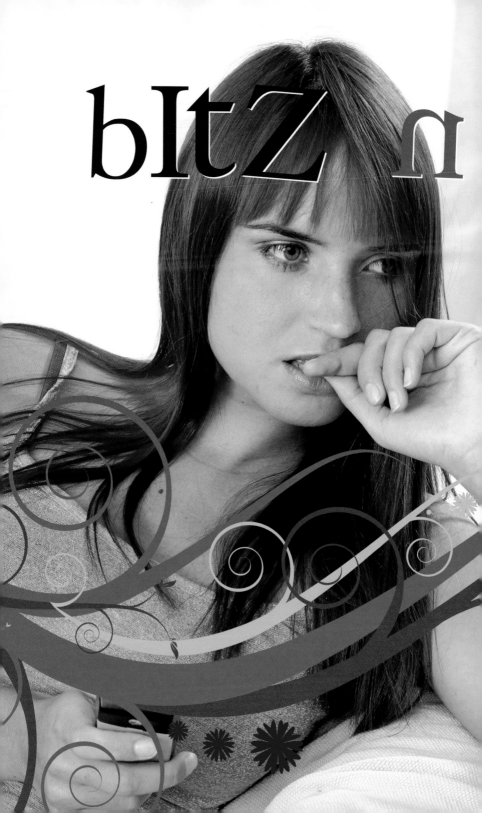

pieces

Now that you've been hit over the head with the news, let's get down to business. I've got something to share with you, something you need very much right about now.

First you have to get past your emotional reaction. Let's concentrate on the positive aspects of your healing. I am not a doctor. Everything I know about chemotherapy has come from my clients. I've asked them to share their feelings about what they have experienced. I have listened and learned.

There is one major truth that outshines all others. A positive attitude brings positive results. Taking time now to understand the process and your options clearly, objectively, with an open mind, will assure successful results. Do yourself this favor.

I realize the huge role hair plays in our image of ourselves. So I understand that now, of all times, you need to look like yourself. When you look good, you feel good. I'm going to explain everything you need to know about wigs to make it through this sensitive time *Looking Like You*.

One of the most satisfying results of my work has been watching so many pleased clients confidently stride out of the salon wearing a smile (and their new hair replacement), looking and feeling so much better than when they arrived.

Many came to me because they saw someone in their support group or at a clinic wearing a beautiful wig I had personalized. Among those who have sought my help are many oncologists and other specialists. Impressed by my simplified explanation of this complex chemical process and my approach to hair replacement, they continue to refer their patients to our shop because of the excellent results my staff and I consistently achieve.

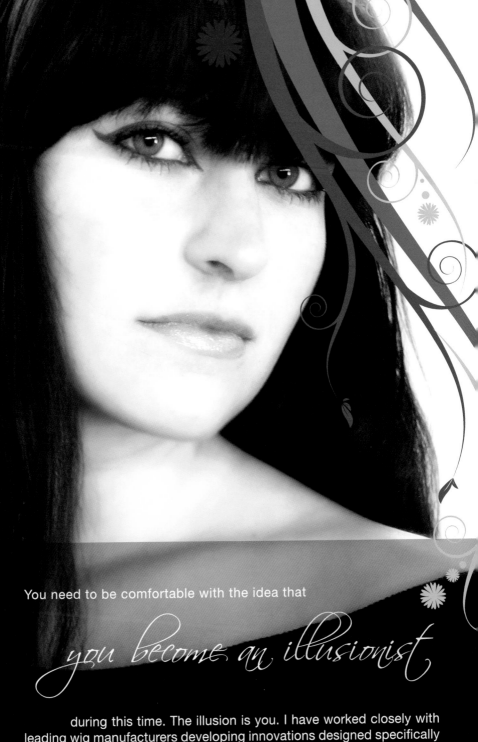

You need to be comfortable with the idea that

you become an illusionist

during this time. The illusion is you. I have worked closely with leading wig manufacturers developing innovations designed specifically with you in mind.

One of the most satisfying results of my work has been watching so many pleased clients confidently stride out of the salon wearing a smile.

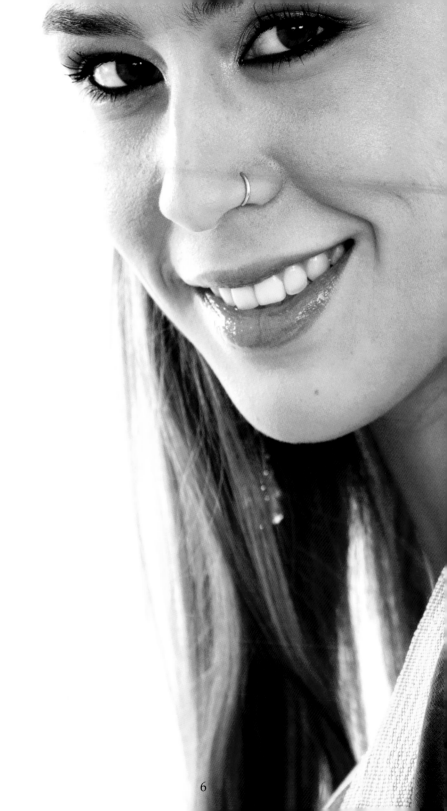

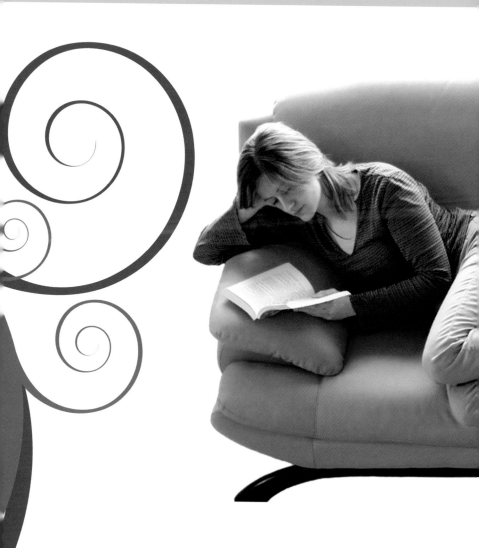

Throughout each chapter, and in a gallery at the end, I've included a sampling of today's latest styles. These have special features you need for your comfort and security. You will learn about basic concepts of design and construction to help you find the perfect wig for you.

With all the how-to's of care, helpful hints, and answers to the most frequently asked questions, you'll feel like an expert! Once your own hair has started growing again, we'll talk about the transition from illusion back to reality.

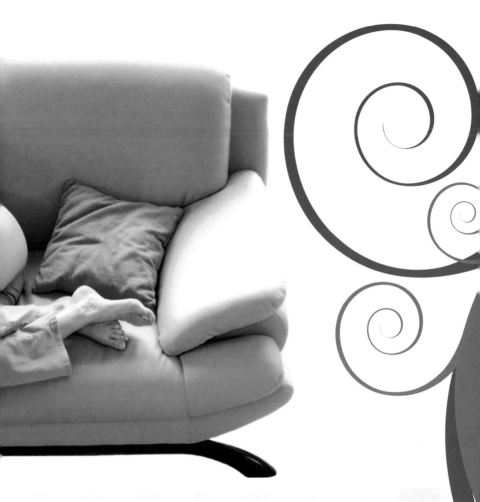

"Read all the way through.
You need to know all of this,
every word."

Read all the way through. You need to know all of this, every word.
You should understand the entire process before you go any further.
I've given this consultation a thousand times. It works again and
again and it's going to work for you!

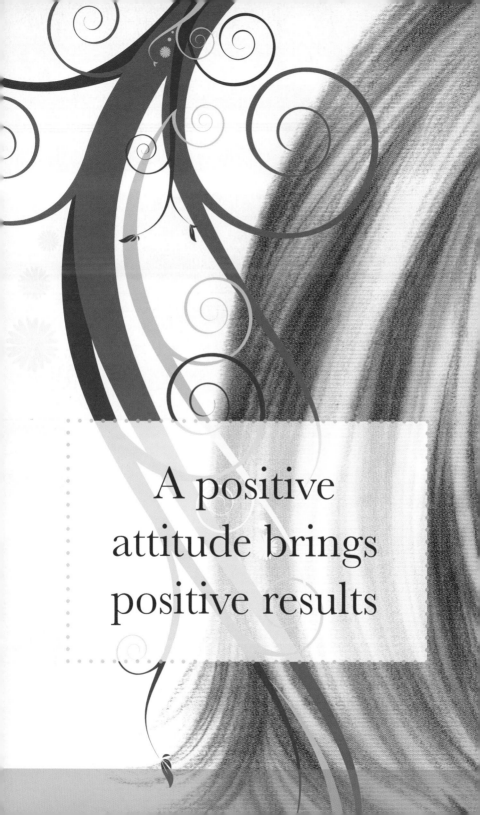

A positive attitude brings positive results

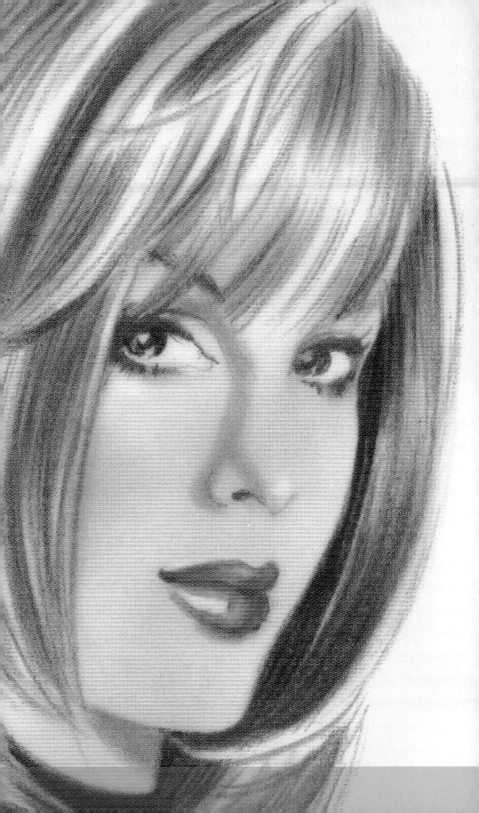

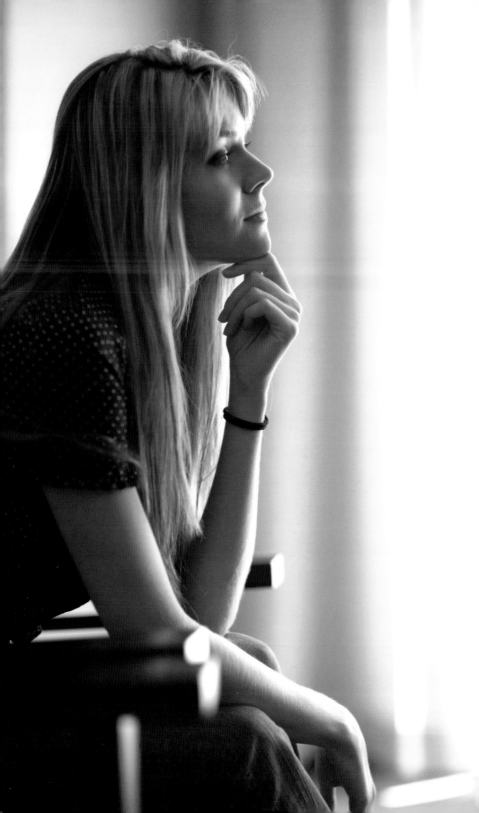

You Need To Know

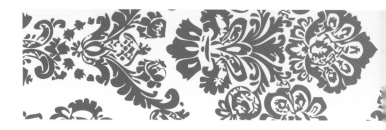

When you first hear you're going to lose your hair as a result of chemotherapy treatments, you can't imagine how it happens. Most people think it falls out all at once or that the treatments kill the hair follicle. Some seem more worried about their looks than the cure.

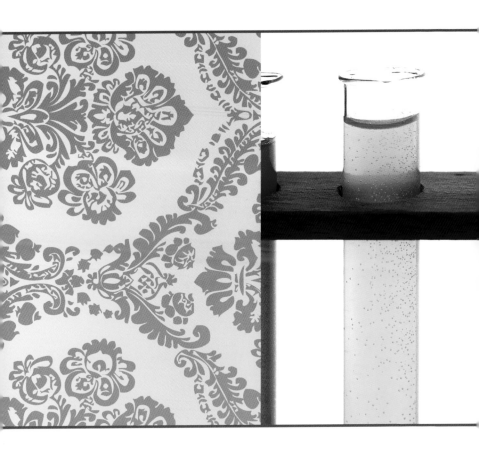

"I have found that taking the time to understand clearly how this complex chemical process works will help enormously in getting past your initial emotional reaction."

As the chemicals used in treatments are absorbed into your system, they begin to affect the cells that make up your entire body. These cells reproduce daily. Every cell is affected including the lymph, saliva, and sinus glands, even the tear ducts, and alas, your hair follicle.

The hair follicle is an egg-shaped cell that has two main functions: to grow hair and to hold the hair shaft in place. When the cells stop dividing, or reproducing, the follicle goes into a sleep like phase. Hair is released from the follicle because the tiny "muscle" that holds the shaft into your scalp

13

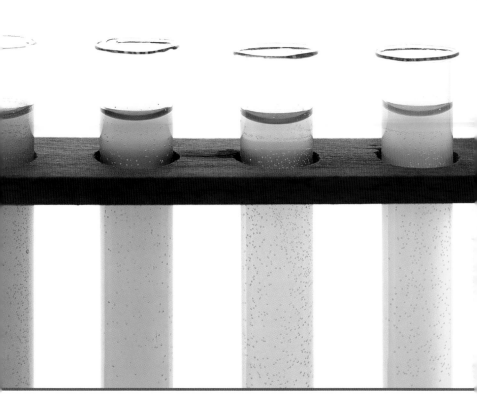

also goes to sleep. The hair simply leaves the scalp. I call it releasing, because that's really all it is.

The hair starts releasing gradually. This doesn't happen all at once. It can take a full week or more for all of the hair to be released. The release usually begins about two weeks after the first treatment, or the week of the second treatment, depending on the medication.

Because cancer is an uncontrolled multiplication of cells, most treatments aggressively combat cell division. The result is complete hair loss. Some courses of treatment may be less intensive. However, it is essential to understand the accumulative nature of these types of treatments.

Be aware that as treatment progresses, the chemicals can build up in your system. Depending on the type of treatment, the chemical buildup may take more or less time. When your body has absorbed a certain level of chemicals, the hair follicle will relax. Whether that is during the second or last week of treatment depends on how aggressive your treatment is.

Talk to your physician who can help you understand which treatment you will be taking and all of its side effects.

There are different reactions to hair release. Some people feel nothing at all. Some feel a slight tingling sensation or experience an over sensitized scalp. Usually reactions stop when the hair has finished releasing.

The chemical treatments can be very dehydrating. To counteract this effect, it is important to drink as much fluid as you can. Water works best for rehydration. When you drink a lot of water, you flush the chemicals from your system. Remember, this is probably the single most important tip anyone could give you for your comfort.

The taste buds also are affected by chemotherapy. The chemicals used tend to leave a metallic taste in your mouth, which can put you off your favorite foods and drinks. If water tastes unpleasant to you, try different brands of bottled water. Each comes from a different part of the world and contains different minerals.

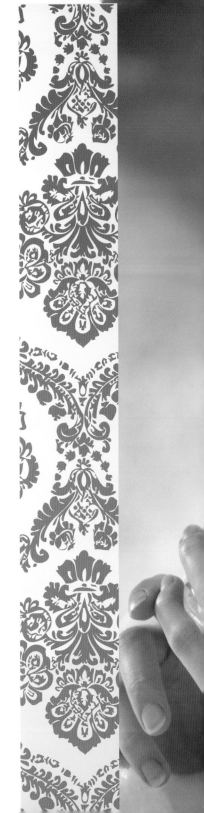

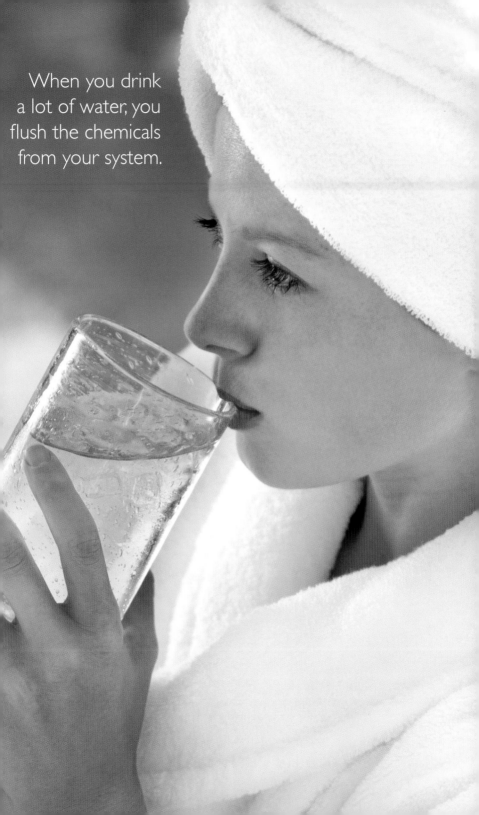

When you drink
a lot of water, you
flush the chemicals
from your system.

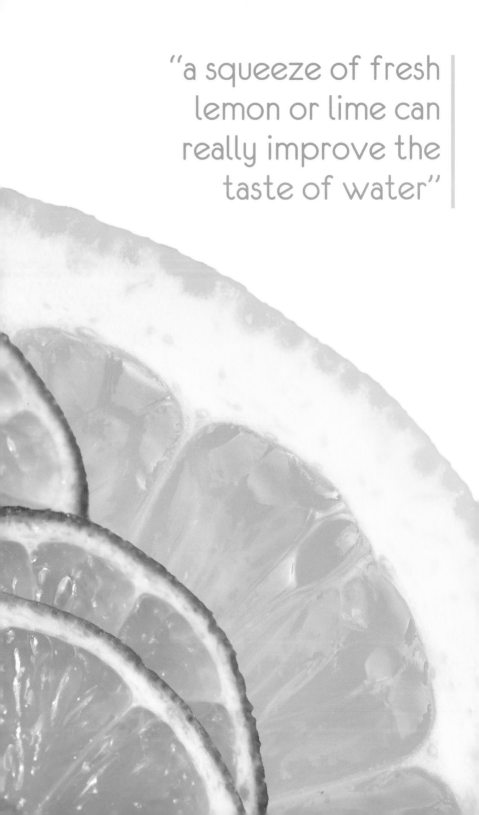

"a squeeze of fresh lemon or lime can really improve the taste of water"

For added refreshment, a squeeze of fresh lemon or lime can really improve the taste of water. My clients have shared other helpful hints. Ice cold sparkling water and soda crackers seem to help with nausea. Chinese green tea is soothing also. It is said to possess healing qualities, according to traditional Chinese medicine.

Here are two more "hints". Carry water or your favorite drink with you wherever you go and get in the habit of constantly sipping. Don't wait until you are thirsty! Those who have a hard time drinking enough water may find they have low energy. It can become a chore to do even the simplest things. Water acts like a charge and gives you energy.

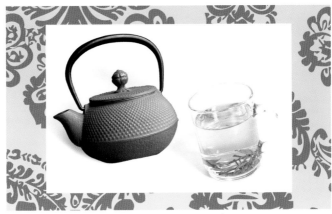

Chinese green tea

Finding the delicate balance between facing reality and creating it can work miracles in healing mind, body, and soul.

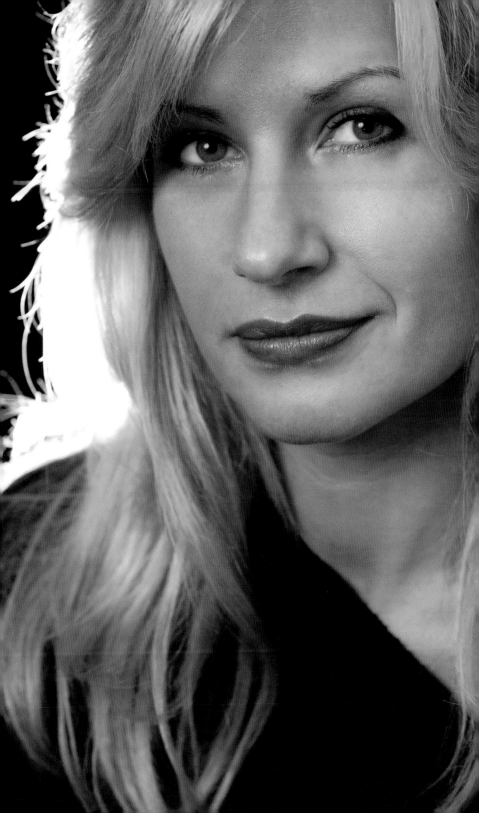

Positive feelings of hope and optimism play a vital role in marshalling all your strength to fight your cancer and handle your chemotherapy. Finding the delicate balance between facing reality and creating it can work miracles in healing mind, body, and soul.

Be open to new possibilities, the right look can work wonders. Today's leading wig styles are truly ready to wear. Additional layering to create wisps of fringe can frame and enhance your facial shape.

The length and angle of your wig's cut can elongate or soften your features, bringing out your best.

I always recommend that you go wig shopping before you start your treatments. This enables your stylist to see your own hair texture, style and color. The tone-on-tone colorings available in ready to wear wigs are amazingly lifelike.

You might want to add custom personalizing. For those with distinctive coloring, adding accents

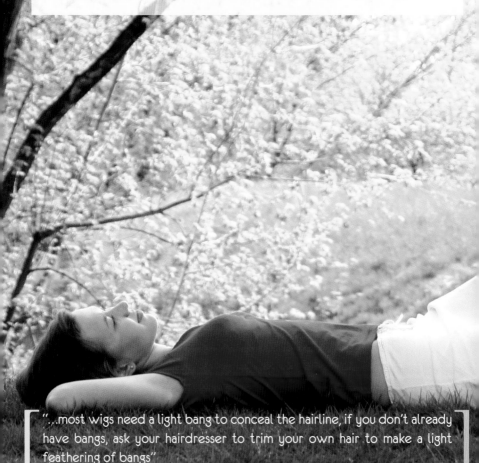

"...most wigs need a light bang to conceal the hairline, if you don't already have bangs, ask your hairdresser to trim your own hair to make a light feathering of bangs"

of color or highlights in the area framing the face often achieves the desired first impression. This can help give quite a natural look.

If you cut your hair short because someone tells you that this will make it easier to handle the hair loss, you'll have two things to deal with: a new change of hairstyle and the new look and feel of a wig. I believe that if you hold off on the haircut and try to make your new wig closely resemble the hairstyle you are comfortable with, you will have better results.

Since most wigs need a light bang to conceal the hairline, if you don't already have bangs, ask your hairdresser to trim your own hair to make a light feathering of bangs. Think of this as an update to your look. It's better to do this before you start wearing the wig. That way no one will notice when you make the switch.

Looking Like You is very important at this time.

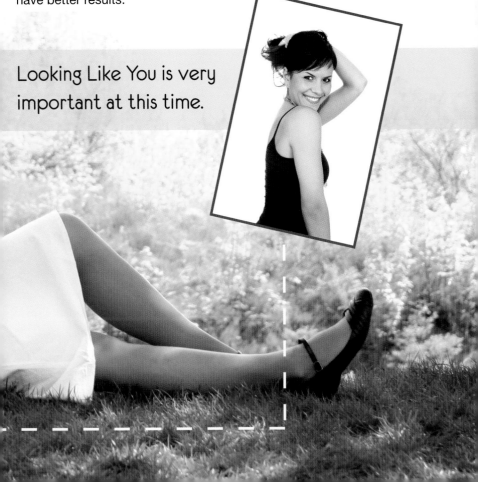

After selecting your hair replacement, don't wait too long to return to your wig stylist. He or she can help you. At our salon, we suggest that you set up an appointment with the stylist when your hair first begins releasing. *This will be your second fitting.* The week your hair starts reacting to the treatments, stop over brushing and discontinue shampooing.

When your hair starts coming out, it is best to remove it. This may seem like a harsh measure, but waiting until it all falls out can be even more traumatic. Deciding when to remove your hair allows you to maintain control. You make the choice. We like to work with the client at this time and offer her this service.

This is when your wig will be sized for comfort. Think of sizing as customizing the fit. Several sets of measurements are taken. Even though ready to wear wigs are adjustable with a stretch fit, in some instances, wefts of hair can be removed in strategic spots. Tabs may be slightly resituated and the circumference tightened or loosened as needed. Sizing the cap results in the perfect fit, snug but not too tight. Once the scalp is bare, *you can secure your wig by using double sided tape.* With this method your wig will not slip or fall off.

Synthetic wigs should never be cut or styled before sizing because this changes the shape of the inside of the cap, which in turn affects the precut style. Its best to have your wig cut and styled after it's been sized. When you make the switch to wearing the wig, no one will notice. You can leave the salon with your wig on... *Looking Like You.*

Your own hair will begin to grow back about two or three weeks after your treatment ends. It will take approximately **six months** for your hair to fill in sufficiently to style on its own. *After one or two months of growth, it's time to stop using tape to secure your wig.* Change to a lock-and-release clip. These clips are sewn onto the tape pads to hold your wig securely.

The hair clip opens and closes by bending and pressing the edges in or out from the center. If you've never seen or used one before, we reccomend you open and close the clip several times to feel and see how the teeth of the clip open and close. It's a snap, and holds the hairpiece in place securely and comfortably.

It is best to shift the positioning of the clips every so often to avoid damaging your new hair as it grows in. Simply remove the clip, reposition it slightly, then re-stitch the clip so your hair is not over stressed in any one spot. This will be more comfortable for you.

Most doctors advise that you avoid hair coloring for the first few months while your hair is growing back. You may instead try a temporary vegetable-based rinse to brighten or enhance your own color. If this kind of rinse only lasts between shampoos, you must re-apply after each shampoo.

When your hair has sufficiently filled in around the nape of your neck, a partial hairpiece will give you just the touch of fullness you'll need. The perfect solution to add volume to fine and thinning hair, integrated hairpieces are ideal for the transitional period while your hair is growing back.

Human hair partials can be colored,

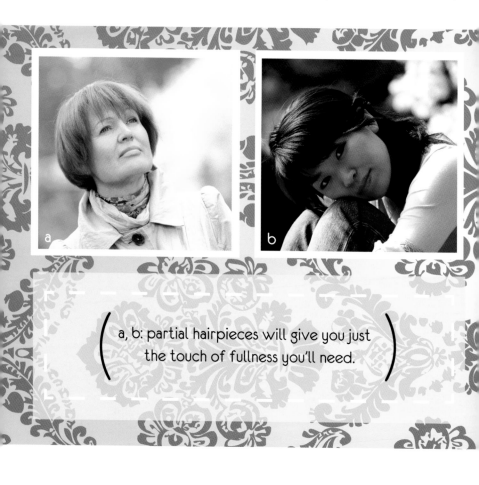

a, b: partial hairpieces will give you just the touch of fullness you'll need.

curled, or permed. Whether you want to add length or just fullness, the latest innovative partial integrated hairpieces are the easiest way to achieve the look. These can become a valuable part of your fashion wardrobe for years to come.

Many clients who were reluctant at first, came to adore the convenience and ease, not to mention fabulous look of their hair replacement. We have actually had to gently nudge them back in the direction of styling their own hair.

At first, almost everyone feels "the whole world knows I have a wig on." In fact, a properly fitted and styled wig is really hard to detect. It's still you…only better.

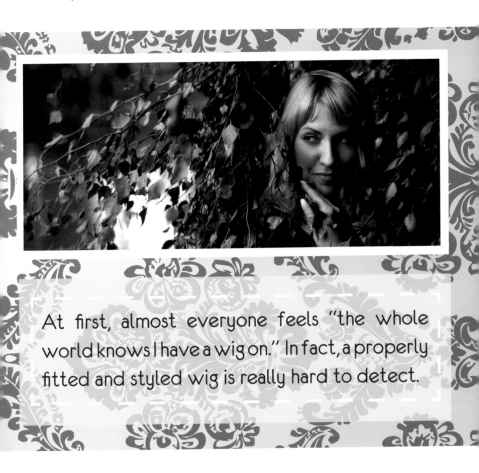

At first, almost everyone feels "the whole world knows I have a wig on." In fact, a properly fitted and styled wig is really hard to detect.

Be open to new
possibilities, the
right look can
work wonders

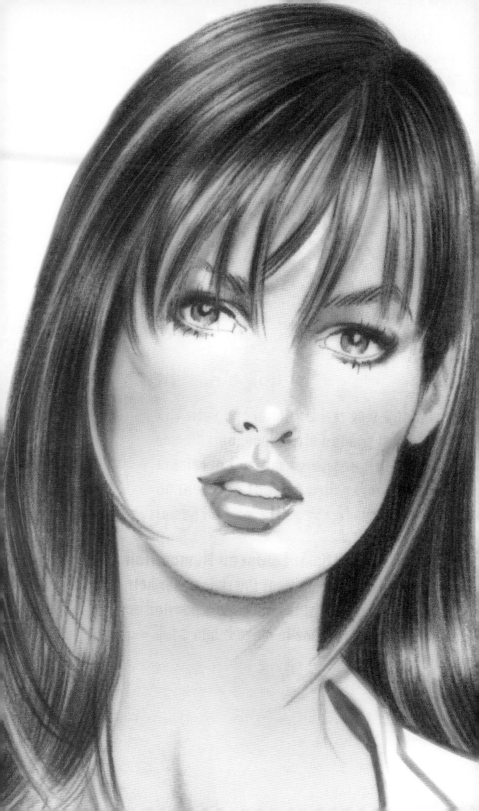

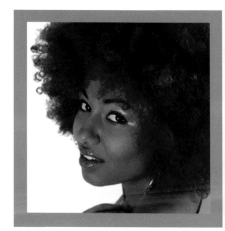
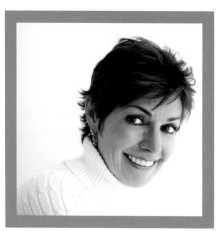

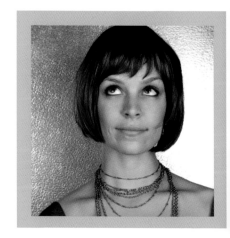

FINDING THE PERFECT WIG

Choosing the right wig for your personal needs is very important. Take it one step at a time. The first step is to understand your options clearly. This will require your full attention. Concentrating on solutions can be a marvelous distraction from the unpleasant side effects of your cure, and that's a good thing!

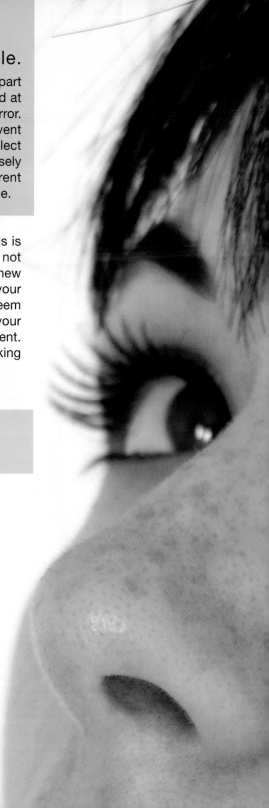

Keep it simple.

Your hairstyle is a significant part of the image you have arrived at over a lifetime of trial and error. Now is not the time to reinvent the wheel. You want to select the hairpiece that most closely resembles your own current color, texture, length and style.

Obvious as it may sound, this is the key to success. This is not the best time to try out a new hair color or style. Changing your hairstyle or coloring may seem like fun, but remember your focus is your hair replacement. The object is to continue Looking Like You.

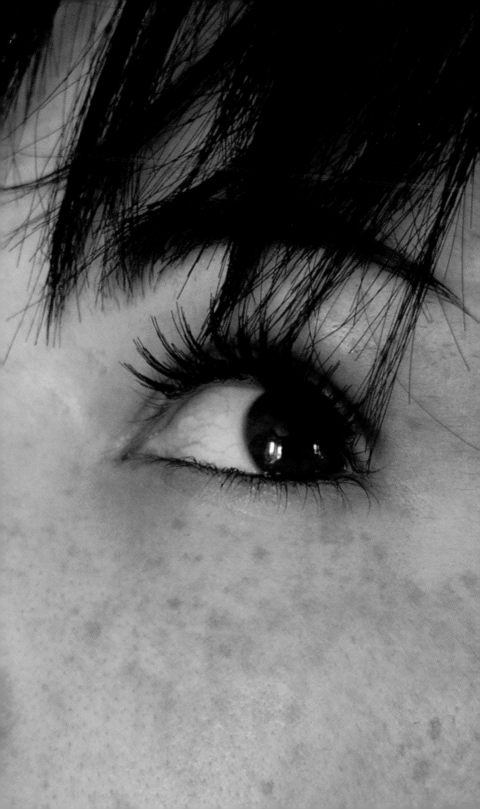

Think of your

new look

as an *update*

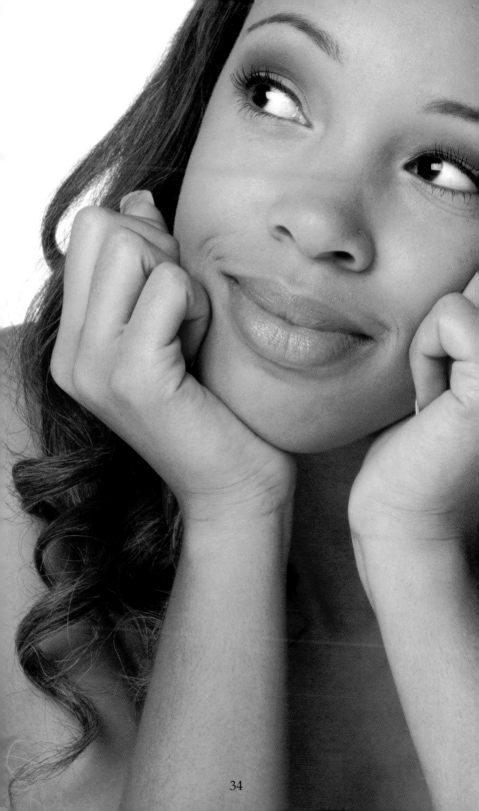

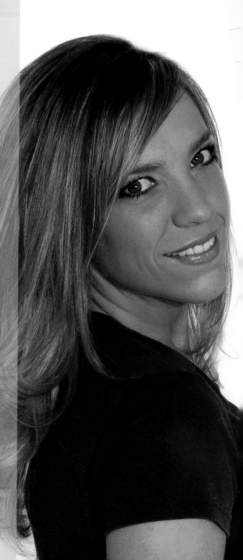

Over time, embrace refinements to your look that may be helpful as your situation changes. Remember, you are solution oriented. Any look, no matter how comfortable and familiar, can use an occasional update. Now is as good a time as any to make certain that your hairstyle is the most flattering to your features. You want to look up to date.

You may find it helpful to take a friend along to assist with selecting the color and style of your new hair. But don't allow too many people to join you. Too many opinions will confuse you, making your selection more difficult.

Trust your stylist to guide you

Bring along a photo of yourself wearing the hairstyle with which you feel most comfortable, or tear pages out of magazines with pictures that closely resemble the style you prefer.

Today's wigs have special features to make them easier than ever to wear. Understand which types will offer you not only the correct style but also added comfort.

There are basically two types of wigs available: *Ready to wear and Custom made.*

Careful attention to a few all-important details will enable you to make your selection with success and ease:

☑ Be positive and attentive.

☑ Keep everything simple and concise.

☑ Become informed to understand your options more clearly.

☑ Ask questions.

☑ Think of your new look as an update.

☑ If this becomes a challenge, exercise patience and persistence.

A positive attitude will bring positive results, always, in all things.

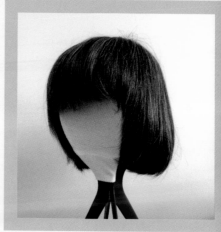

Today's state-of-the-art wigs are offered in a wide variety of current chic modern styles in every coloring. There are three types of ready to wear wigs available: natural hair, synthetic fiber and blends. Blends are a mixture of real hair with synthetic fiber. Wigs are either handmade or machine made or a combination of both. The combination of machine made with handmade features is the latest innovation in ready-to-wear.

The handmade mono filament top is a wonderful recent innovation. We call this the "breathing cap" because it is so lightweight.

Strand by strand the hair is sewn onto a transparent nylon netting. When placed on bare skin, the hair appears to be growing right out of the scalp. This feature is similar in appearance to custom wigs.

Most of these wigs have a machine-made stretch back to assure the best fit. Since everyone's head has a shape unique to that person, today's wig cap is detailed with adjustable velcro tabs that can be easily adjusted to conform to your head.

These natural looking wigs now are available in human hair as well as synthetic, or a blend of real with synthetic fiber.

The latest innovation is natural virgin hair with the cuticles intact, guaranteed not to tangle.

Because of their quality, mono-filament wigs are a little more expensive than regular machine made styles. Real hair is priced higher while synthetics tend to be less expensive.

READY TO WEAR

With recent developments in synthetic fiber, these wigs are remarkably natural in texture. Differences in synthetic fibers come from the thickness. Fiber with a greater thickness is used for straighter styles. Thinner fiber is used for creating soft curly textures. A mixture of these fibers may be used to achieve the desired effect.

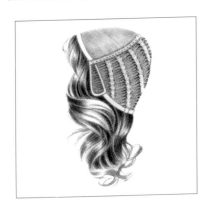

Professional stylists will understand your type of curl pattern and texture. Curl patterns in hair or fiber occur in "s" shaped curves. In wig making these s-waves are tighter or more relaxed to produce the degree of curl. So a short bob uses a thicker fiber for a straighter look. A soft curly style would employ thinner fiber with a more condensed s-wave. Many styles are best achieved by altering the curl pattern in certain areas where extra fullness is desirable.

Blends use synthetic fiber for styling support added to real hair. These offer the most attractive and practical option for many of today's popular hairstyles.

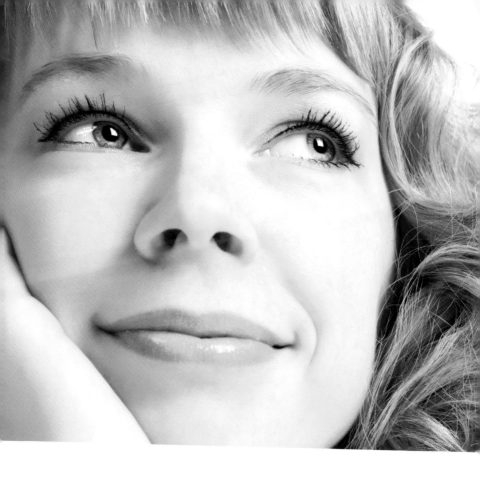

Many of today's leading wig styles are truly ready to wear as they are. But you may want to take it from there, adding custom personalization to your ready to wear wig. In styling, additional layering to create wisps of fringe will frame and enhance your facial shape.

A square face shape could round out the forehead with fringe and soften the jaw line with layering. A diamond face shape, with wide cheekbones, might benefit from fullness at the jaw line. The length and angle of your wig's cut can elongate or soften your

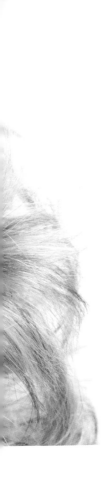

features, framing and flattering your facial shape. You want to accentuate the positive, bringing out your best attributes.

There are lifelike blends of colorings, tone-on-tone, to match almost anyone's natural or enhanced hair color. For those with distinctive coloring, adding accents of color or highlights in the area framing the face will often achieve the desired first impression.

Some find that one wig is sufficient for their particular needs during this time. If this is the case, careful attention to the details of your maintenance strategy will pay off nicely. Once you are comfortable with the style and fit of either a custom or ready-to-wear, we find that it is the most practical option to order a back-up. You may choose to have an exact duplicate, or perhaps a less expensive alternate for more casual wear, or both.

This enables you to freshen up your look quickly. If you've worn your wig all day and then want to have an evening on the town, you can simply change into a fresh one.

Alternating your wigs in this manner allows more wear between restyling. This way you can wear one while the other is being cleaned. Also, in the event of damage or loss, you'll always be prepared, which is never a bad idea.

Body heat eventually will stretch the elastic in the foundation. With the strenuous activities of everyday life, prolonged wear changes the texture of synthetic fiber. Even the finest of wigs worn daily, will, after a period of time, begin to show wear and tear.

A mono-filament top gives a lifelike scalp

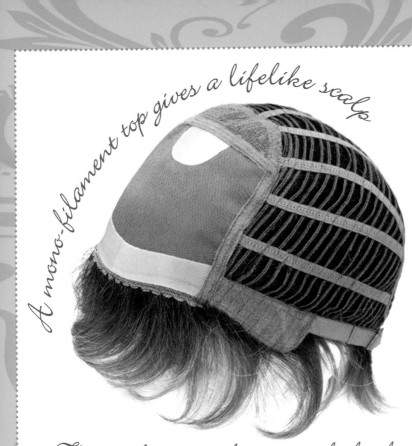

The capless machine-made back breathes and is so comfortable

Easy adjustment tabs assure the perfect fit

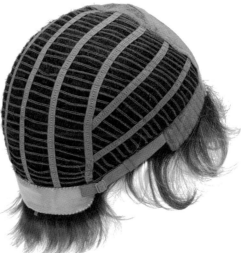

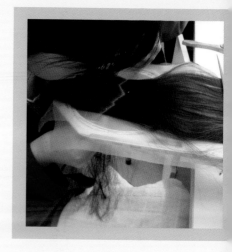

Highly skilled wigmakers have created magnificent hairpieces in much the same manner for centuries. Custom handmade wigs are widely used in theater and film for the remarkably lifelike effect they achieve. They are also very popular as a fashion accessory for special occasions. Every woman has a highly personal style unique to her. To duplicate your exact hairstyle to your unique specifications you may order a custom handmade wig in either human hair or synthetic.

Look for the wigmakers who can show you examples of their work before you place your order. This will show you the kind of workmanship you can expect. Custom wig making requires at least four to six weeks, so be sure to allow enough time to prepare.

Make it clear that you want the finished product to resemble your own hairstyle. When making special requests, clearly identify and communicate any personal characteristics you are looking for. This may be a streak of color, or a wave in a particular area.

Whether it's human hair or synthetic, you want to match color, texture, thickness, and the curl pattern of your hair. If you want a perfect match, it is always best to provide a swatch of your own hair.

Hair has different characteristics depending upon its origin. European hair is used because of its natural wave and sheen. Asian hair is stronger and more durable and can be permed or processed.

CUSTOM MADE

For many years wigs were mostly made from Asian hair. Indian hair tends to have a fine silky texture. Wigmakers use each for its particular textural advantage. All hair to be used should be shown to you for your approval before the wigmaker begins making your hairpiece.

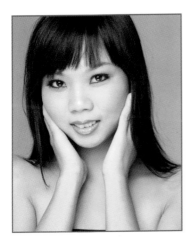

Choosing natural hair allows an exact match to your own texture and color. There are two types of hair available for wig making, virgin and descaled. Virgin European hair still has its cuticle. It posses a wonderful luster and color as well as its natural curl pattern. Virgin European hair is one of the softest hair. Descaled hair has the cuticle removed by a chemical process to keep it from tangling when washed. Descaled hair is straighter hair and often used to blend with other types of hair to produce a softer quality refined hair or European texture.

A variety of lightweight durable materials may be used to create a super light airy cap for your comfort. Gauze, netting, and mono filament, or a combination of these are constructed using your exact measurements. Circumference, over the head, ear to ear, and distance from the nape of the neck to the hairline are carefully measured. The desired result is a perfect fit, snug but not too tight. Pre-made caps also are available. It is important that you make sure your cap fits before the hair is added.

After you have approved the hair to be used, it is added to the cap by the art of ventilating.

Ventilating is the process of knotting a few strands at a time with a special needle, very much like crocheting. Ventilating gives the most natural life-like head of hair, because it allows the wigmaker to have complete control of thickness. The ventilator takes a very artistic approach in building a wig from the nape of the neck up to the hairline, creating the exact degree of thickness to achieve the desired look.

Highlights or distinctive areas of color may be added. In some cases a slight graying may be desirable.

Hairlines may be added on very fine almost invisible silk netting called "lace". These are glued to the scalp with water or spirit-based adhesive. This process gives the appearance of hair growing right from your hairline. Wigs with a lace hairline are very delicate and usually require servicing at a salon.

Custom wig making is truly a skill of timeless artistry. Once your wig has been constructed, your appropriate cut and style will be the finishing touch. If you are taking your wig to a stylist other than the wigmaker, make certain the stylist understands the art of styling a custom made wig. Because you have to leave your custom wig for salon maintenance care, it is wise to have a second wig as a backup. When you are satisfied with the fit and style, you may wish to order a duplicate. Or, you may find that a ready to wear wig is a practical choice for your backup.

—

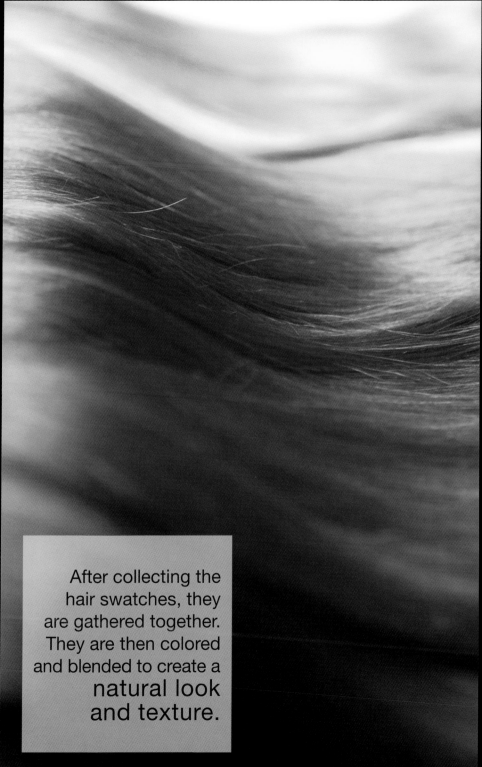

After collecting the hair swatches, they are gathered together. They are then colored and blended to create a **natural look and texture.**

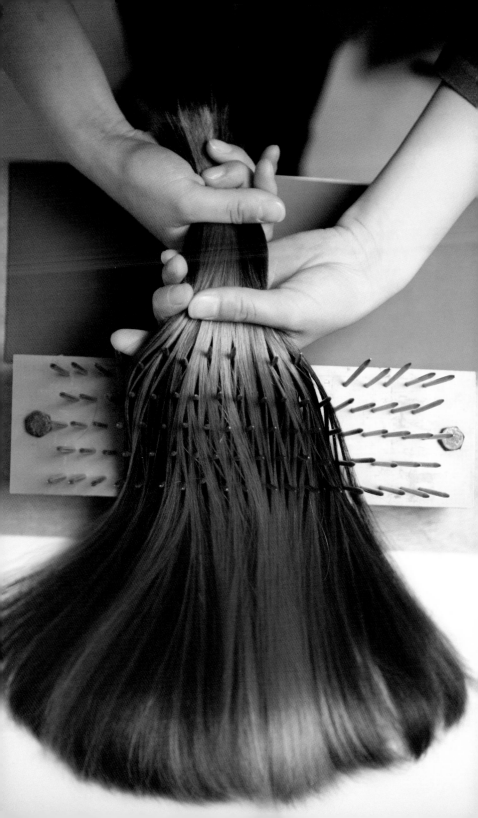

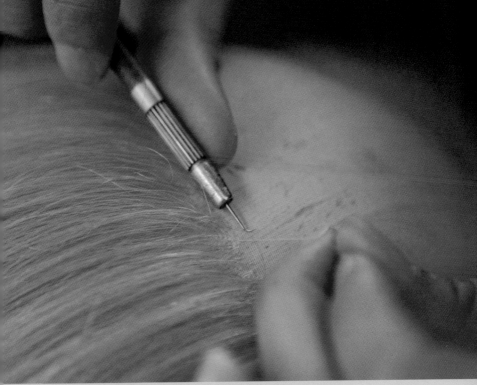

Custom blending and ventilating hair requires skillful handwork and patience.

Each hairpiece takes weeks to create.

Custom measurements assure you the
perfect fit.

Using today's finest natural European hair and lace foundations, custom wigs are the sure way to guarantee the right fit, look and comfort.

Any look, no
matter how
comfortable and
familiar can use an
occasional update.

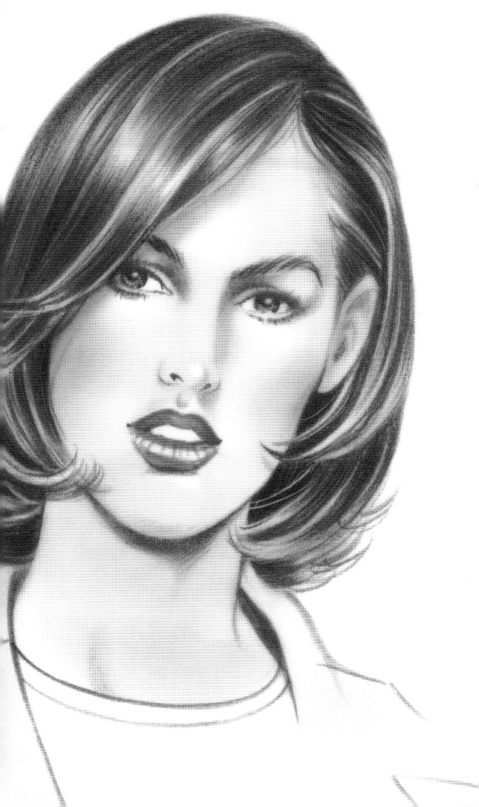

Putting it Together

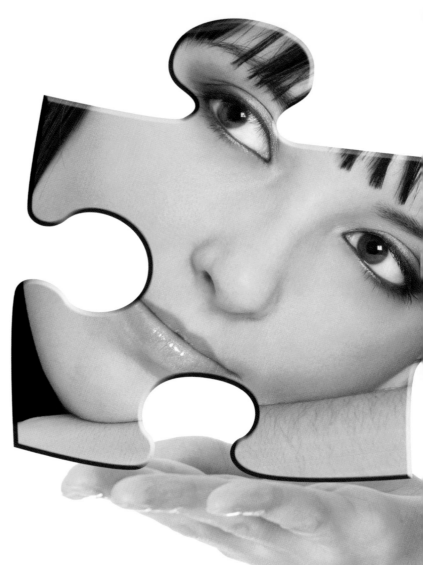

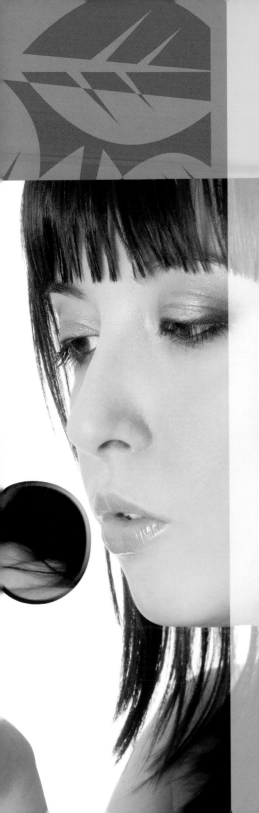

"Putting it together bit by bit, piece by piece"

...like the song says, build an effective strategy right from the start. Now that you're familiar with the different types of wigs, let's review some considerations for the different types of personalities who wear them. You can easily use any of these strategies or styling tips. In the beginning, you should keep it simple. Your main concern is comfort and ease. You can always elaborate later. Employ whatever works for you, and enjoy!

Business women want to convey a clean cut corporate image. Classic basic bobs and short layered wigs work very well for a professional look. Those with longer hair might consider an update with a wig in a more sleek modern style. Think of an efficient cut, which is more easily maintained on the go. An excellent choice for your second piece could be a more casual style. Wear this for relaxing on weekends and evenings, keeping your primary piece ready to go. This pays off big time on hurried workday mornings.

Accents of color are key to dressing for success. You can use all your favorite hair accessories with your wig. Headbands in a narrow width slide onto your wig easily. If the band is too thick it will stick out on the sides. Look for more petite headbands with a serrated edge to hold the band in place. Try tortoise shell, ribbon or suede, and colorful plastic bands. Sparkling glittery ornaments add instant pizzaz for evening.

Barrettes, clip-in bows, and combs add lift to the sides and can come in handy for quick changes after hours. For a fresh easy look at work, clip a few strands up to the side to keep stray hair off your face. Always be mindful of the wig's hairline.

There are more styling options for your wig than you may realize. With longer styles, gently gather the hair at the nape of the neck into a clip comb for a ponytail look. Keep it loose behind the ear area to conceal the hairline. This is a great look for both work and play. Feel free to use your imagination and experiment with fun looks, just like you always have with your own hair.

You can find great butterfly clips of all sizes and combs with elasticized fabrics that are perfect for quick easy styling. A scarf worn around the neck for daytime can later double as a head wrap while exercising. Be prepared for afternoon gym workouts, a walk in the park, whatever. Plan ahead.

When on the go, get into the habit of always checking yourself out in a mirror before arriving for appointments.

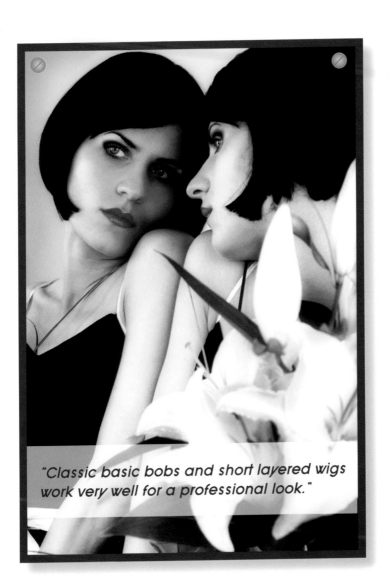

"Classic basic bobs and short layered wigs work very well for a professional look."

Your wig may need a quick retouch.

Just *mist* lightly

and arrange with your fingers.

You want to make your best impression, Looking Like You...

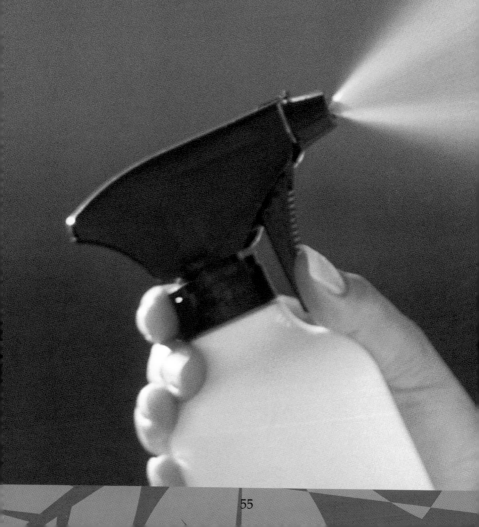

With busy schedules, active moms will want to keep things practical. Any working mother is already an expert at that. With scheduling changes resulting from your treatments, especially where younger family members are involved,

you may find it easiest to stick to the look your children are familiar with

You may want to let your kids in on your secret. Just be reassuring and include them. Some women have the need to not share the details of their hair replacement with their family. With simple planning, the matter can easily remain private.

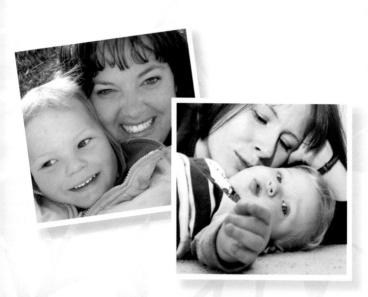

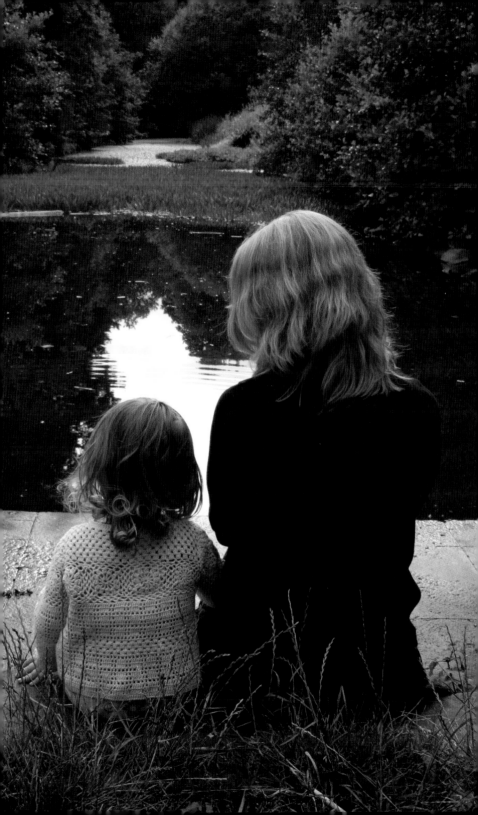

Wigs in a variety of flattering shades, lengths, and styles will add versatility.

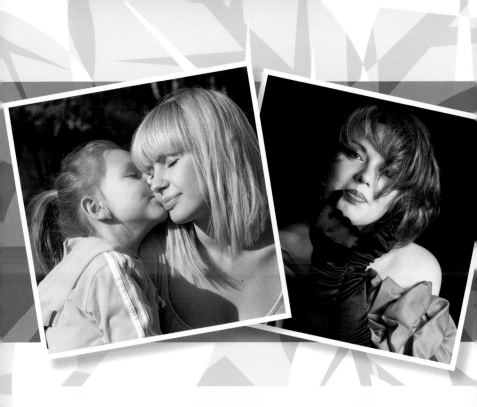

Very young tots have a tendency to grab anything and everything at all times. For playtime with the kids, just take a few more precautions in securing your hairpiece. Add extra tape in a few strategic spots, for a snug fit. Headbands, a bandanna or scarf can help. Also available are fabric head wraps that tie easily.

Your older kids may enjoy accompanying you to the salon. They can be reassuring and assist in making your selections. A grown daughter can be a great help with her sense of current fashion trends. This can become an excellent opportunity for sharing special time together.

Actresses and models may select a wig that closely resembles the headshot in their portfolio. Take this along when shopping for your wig to show your stylist.

Also, you might find it advantageous to discuss your hair replacement strategy with your management or agency. They may be helpful in offering advice to give you the look that will work for you.

Wigs in a variety of flattering shades, lengths, and styles will add versatility. Your collection of hairpieces could include ponytail switches, and falls for added length and glamour. There are brilliant options to explore.

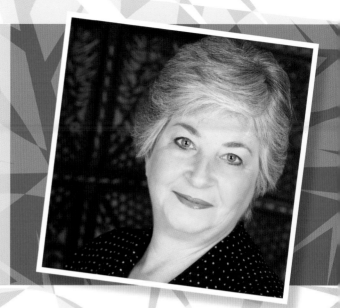

Left to Right:

• let *your* child partake in making the right decision.

• actresses should select a wig that resembes their headshot

• for grey hair. keep it feathered at the crown for a more natural look.

As you age, slightly lighter shades will lift your complexion and brighten your overall appearance.

For silver or white shades try a modern cut. The results can be amazing. If you feel your wig is too full, ask your stylist for their expert opinion. You can easily have your piece professionally feathered and thinned for less volume around your face. Also, a light feathering at the crown will assure a more natural youthful look. This can make a subtle, yet very pleasing difference.

It is also very important to remember that any thinning and feathering should never be attempted until after the cap has been sized to your specifications.

For those with distinctive streaks or areas of color, these special touches are added to their wig by ventilating, in the same manner as a custom wig is created, a few strands at a time. This allows total control of where and how much color is added. Soft pale shades of champagne and blonde may be an option for some. Brunettes may go a few shades lighter for a natural look. Reds and strawberry blondes may also add softer shades for color accents. If your hair has a sprinkling of grey, you may reduce the grey within your color slightly, not totally eliminating a hint of grey. In some cases, a temporary color rinse will work very well in more closely matching your color tone.

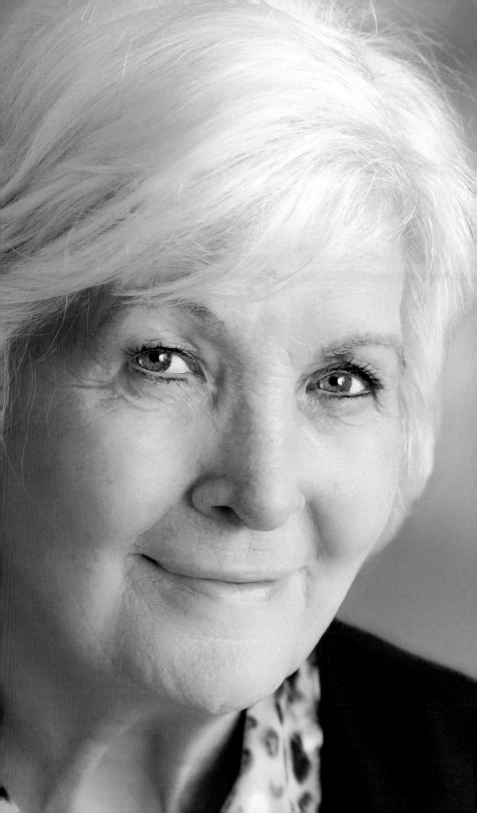

A fashion hint for those with silver or white hair is to wear softly textured sweaters or tops in angora, cashmere, or mohair. These fabrics flatter the texture and color of your hair.

Your best color schemes are monochromatic, like purples with lavender.

Cool blue toned pastels, rather than darker colors, work best around the face. *Avoid colors with a yellow undertone, yellow greens, earth tones, brassy gold or copper jewelry, and rough textures, such as tweed.*

Turbans and head wraps are useful for many occasions. There are 3/4 wigs available in many different lengths that come attached to classic headbands. Attachable bangs, feathered lightly and personalized with highlights, are handy for hats and turbans. Adding just a few simple options can bring a world of variety to your hairpiece collection and spice up your life considerably.

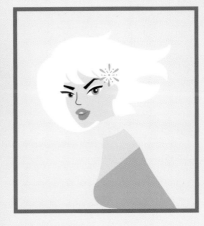

With simple
planning, the
matter can easily
remain private.

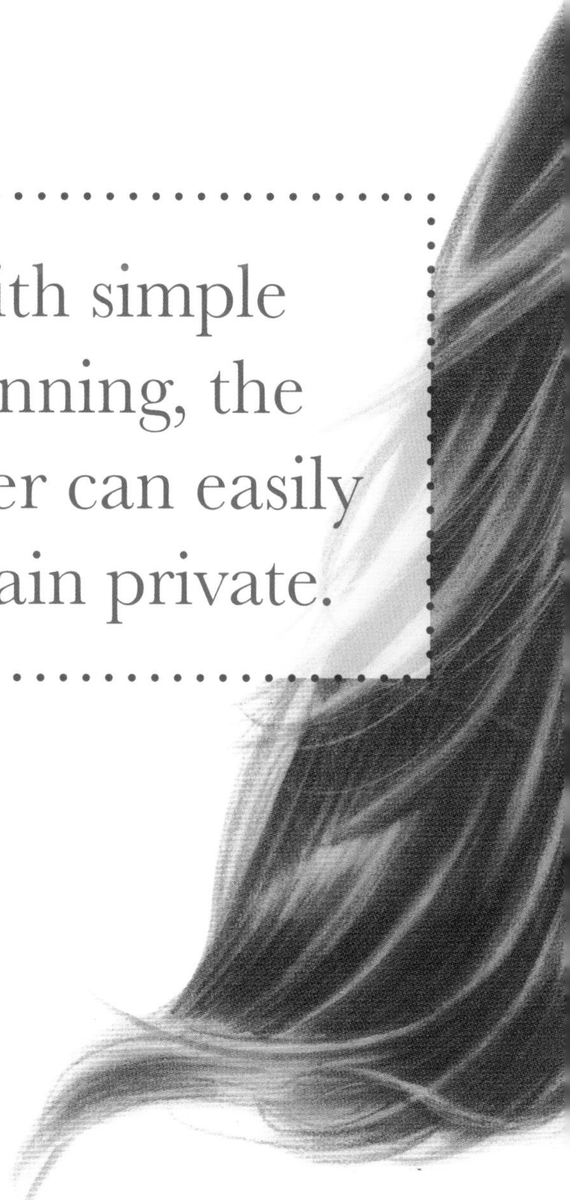

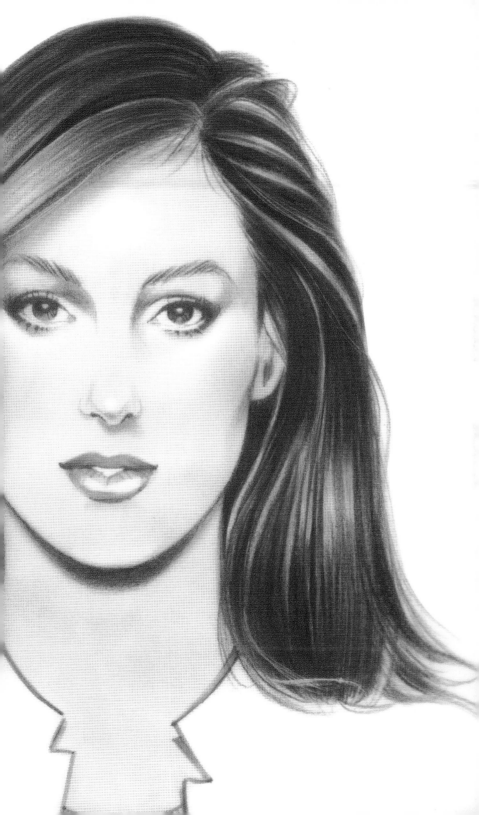

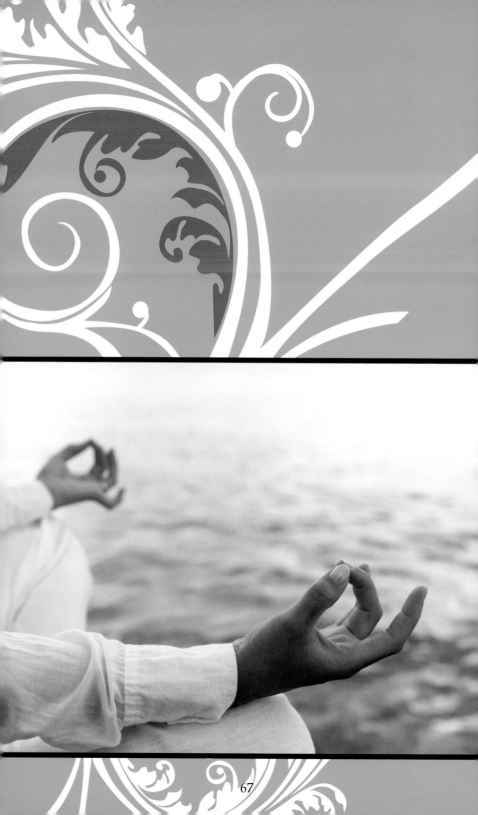

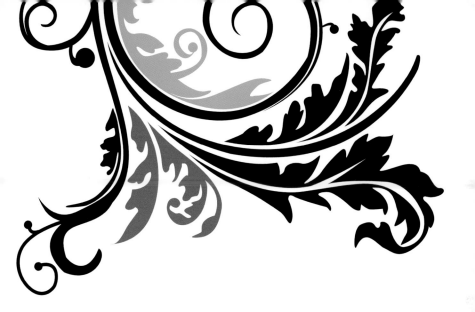

I have some helpful ideas to make it easier to maintain your look even with an active lifestyle. With planning and some simple organization you can be versatile enough to be comfortable in almost every situation, all year round. The more you stick to your normal routine, the better, many doctors advise.

You may enjoy short strolls or long walks, cycling, aerobics, gym workouts, YOGA, tennis, golf, boating, and any of your favorite activities. These keep your spirits bright.

If you want the freedom to exercise, jog, or play a sport, gym options such as cover-ups and head wraps are easy and very trendy. Bandannas work well under baseball caps. Headbands are also great to secure your wig.

The more you stick to your

normal routine,

the better,

many doctors advise.

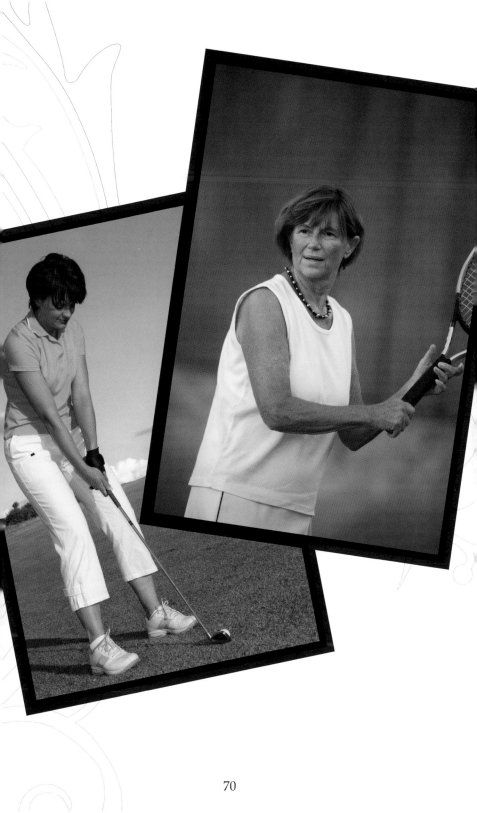

It is always best to avoid getting overheated while wearing your good wig. If you must wear hair at these times, I recommend a less expensive synthetic wig. This will save your better wig from the damaging effects of sweat and excessive body heat. Pace yourself to remain calm, cool, and collected.

There is a chic and modern hairpiece that's the perfect alternative to a full wig for casual or sporty occasions. It consists of a stretch headband with a 3/4 wig attached at the back. Think of this handy option as a fashionable accessory. You can wear it anytime for a fresh active look.

Consider wearing an absorbent turban with attachable bangs, or even solo without any hairpiece, for particularly strenuous workouts.

Leave your wig on its stand while you exercise. After your shower and touching up your face you can replace your hairpiece.

The idea is to make it easier and more convenient to enjoy sports and outdoor fun, as well as certain intimate indoor activities. Treat it as if it's your own hair, it is. The fact that it's a wig is secondary. Feel free to run your fingers through your wig, shake your head, and feel the breeze.

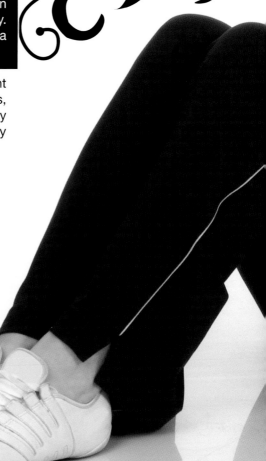

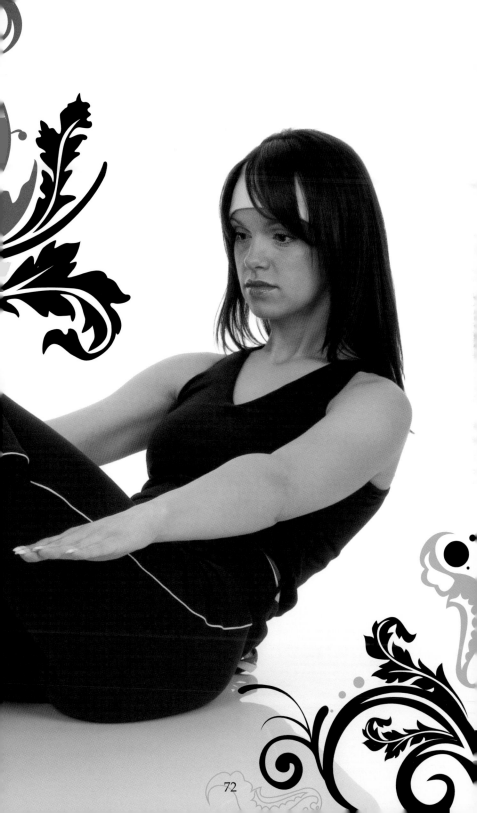

In the words
of a famous
Hollywood stylist,
*"shake your head,
darling!"*

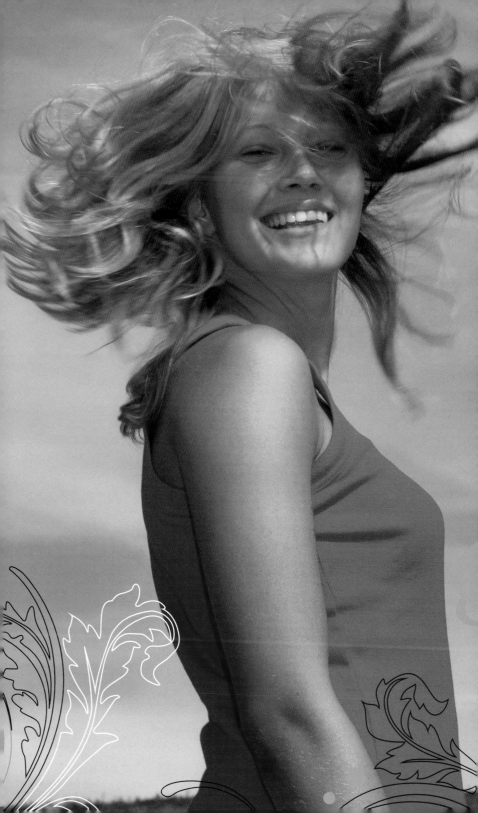

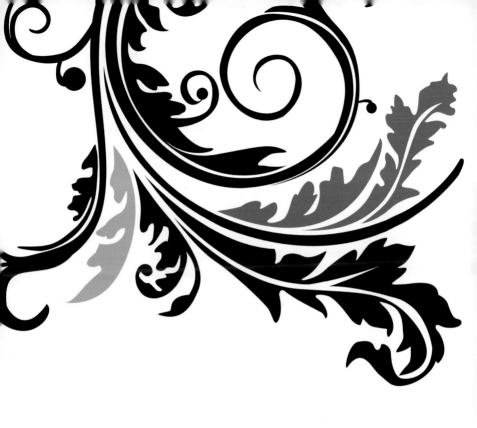

Treat it as if it's your own hair, it is. The fact that it's a wig is secondary.

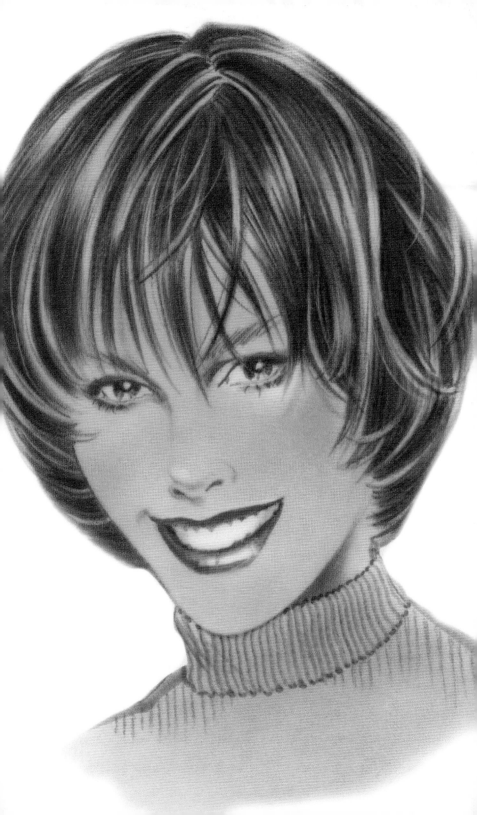

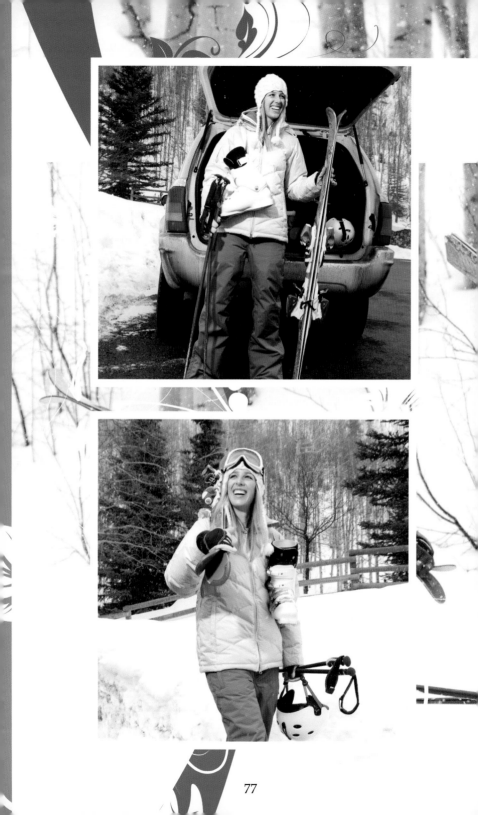

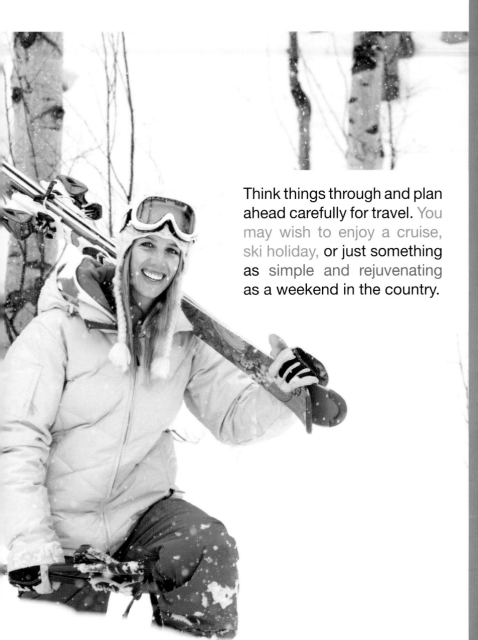

Just in Case

Think things through and plan ahead carefully for travel. You may wish to enjoy a cruise, ski holiday, or just something as simple and rejuvenating as a weekend in the country.

Travel anywhere should first be discussed with your doctor. Make sure to coordinate plans with the timing of your treatment cycles, and medical regime. Once you have the go-ahead, your travel strategy should include hairpieces, essential care items, and adequate accessories.

You want to be prepared for about anything, at all times. Assemble your "just in case" kit, about the size of a makeup bag, for ready access while on the go. Keep it simple, but cover your bases.

Make sure to include a mirror, either a compact or a small lightweight portable with a magnifying side for close-up retouches. *The basics may include extra tape, lock and release clips, needle and thread, small scissors, vent brush, comb with pick, bobby pins, hairspray or mousse, and a small misting bottle.* A chinstrap is used to hold the wig in place while you fluff and brush to refresh your hairstyle. Include this along with a lightweight plastic wig stand for overnighters or whenever you might remove your wig.

For unexpected weather, carry a plastic folding rain cap in your purse. Always be sure to bring this

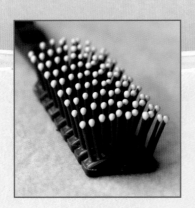
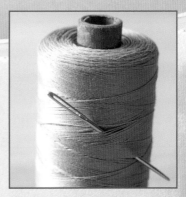
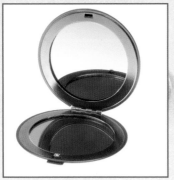
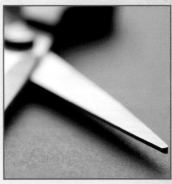

season's neutral versatile scarf, a soft one large enough to double as a head wrap, just in case. Scarves in shiny silky textures tend to slide off the head, so softly coarse textures for headwear are best.

Daytime makeup for a healthy glow is a real perk. For evening, add another coat of mascara, and retouch your brows for dimmer light. A light application of lip balm is invigorating. Add sheer formula lipstick in a richer color, or use lip pencil, making sure never to leave an obvious line, and gloss. A dusting of bronzer or cheek color lightly patted with powdered rice paper for blotting really works to cut shine. Misting sets and gives you a dewy complexion. Carry only the essentials in your kit, to refresh your look quickly and easily anywhere, anytime.

One fashion essential is a pair of sunglasses that flatters your facial shape and hairstyle. Wear your hairpiece when shopping for them. Try a basic classic in neutral or black. Sunglasses are the finishing touch to a chic modern look.

Find a neutral soft leather or wool shoulder bag large enough to accommodate your kit, and other essentials. **Roomy totes are super-functional, and they look sharp with everything all year.**

some of the essentials you should carry with you:

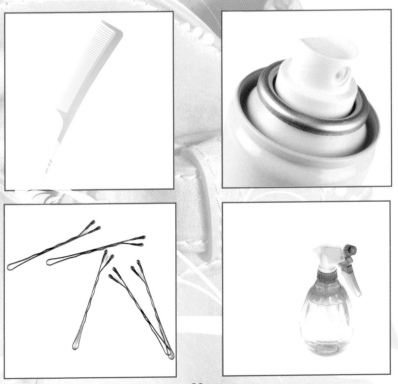

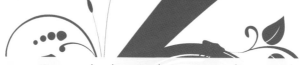

Add sheer formula lipstick in a richer color, or use lip pencil, making sure never to leave an obvious line, and gloss.

A dusting of bronzer or cheek color lightly patted with powdered rice paper for blotting really works to cut shine.

One fashion essential is a pair of sunglasses that flatters your facial shape and hairstyle. Wear your hairpiece when shopping for them. Try a basic classic in neutral or black.

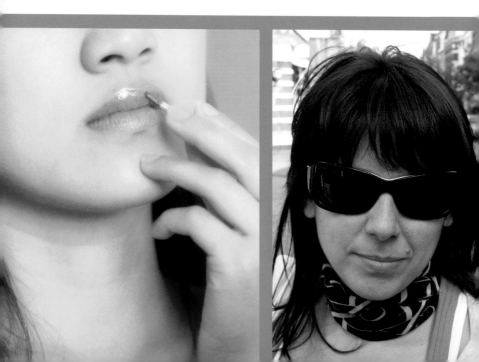

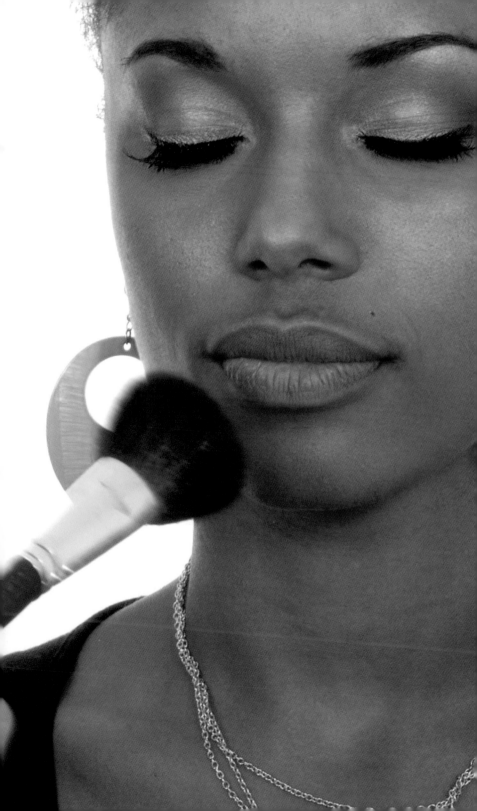

Sunglasses are the finishing touch to a chic modern look.

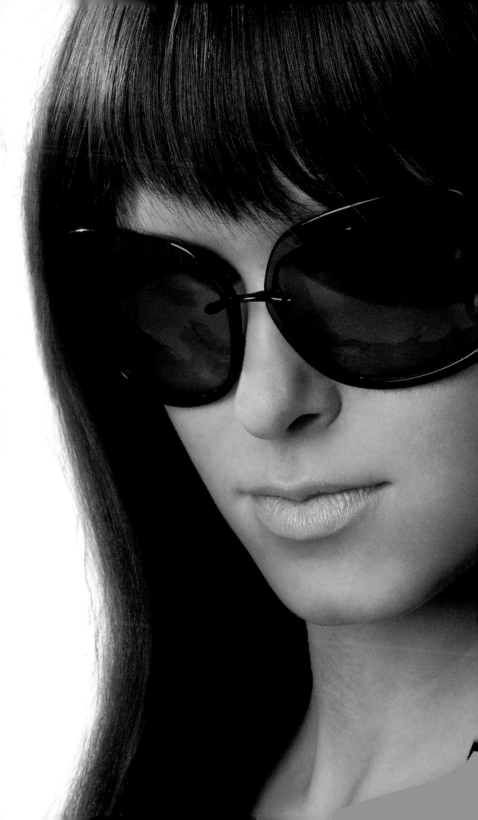

Another must for your kit is a simple basic hat in a crushable fabric that will fit into your shoulder bag. It can be cotton, linen, micro fiber or straw. Just make sure it folds or flattens and still retains its shape. Always allow enough room for your wig to fit under your hat comfortably. When you remove a hat, fluff your wig lightly and mist. Hats that have adequate ventilation in a loose weave are best. A hat worn at a slight angle looks sportier. Hats worn with sunglasses add glamour to any look.

Make sure to always have your latest seasonal options in your kit. They'll be available just when and where you need them. This versatility gives you peace of mind, confidence, and style, Looking Like You...

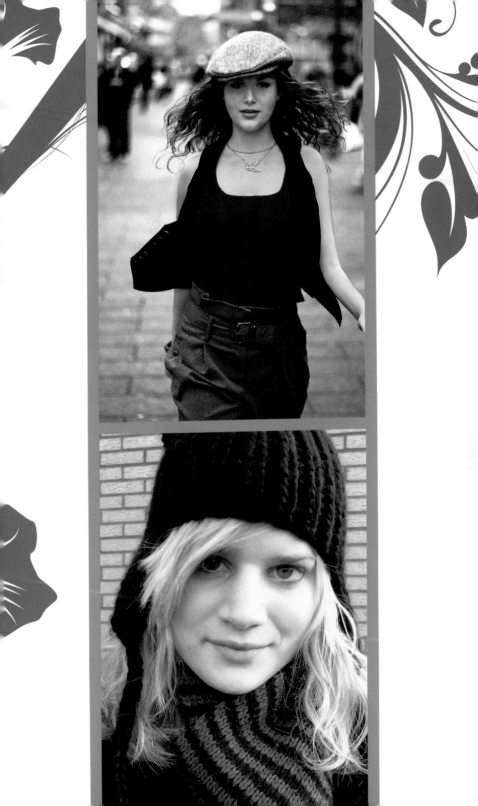

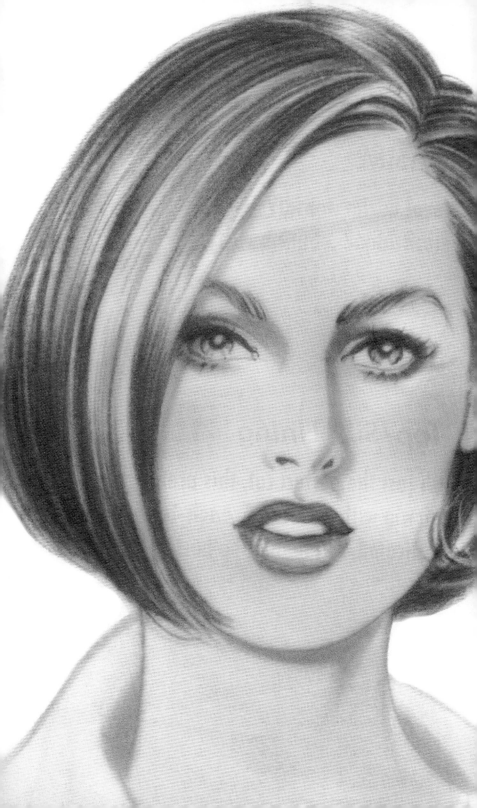

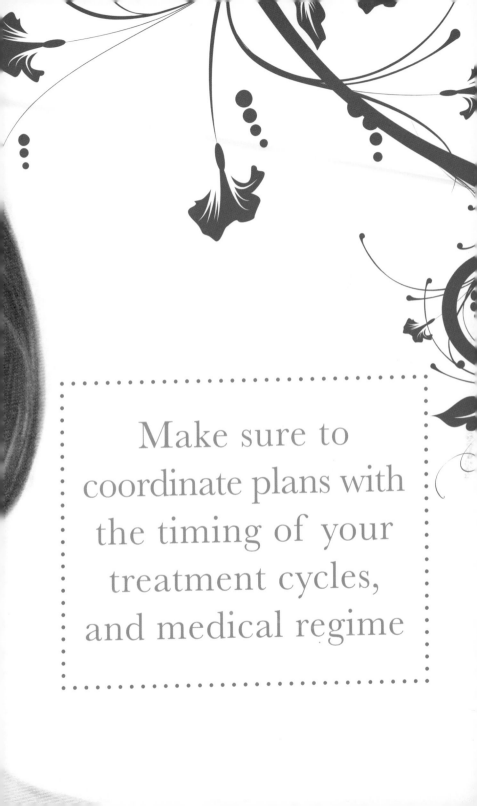

Make sure to coordinate plans with the timing of your treatment cycles, and medical regime

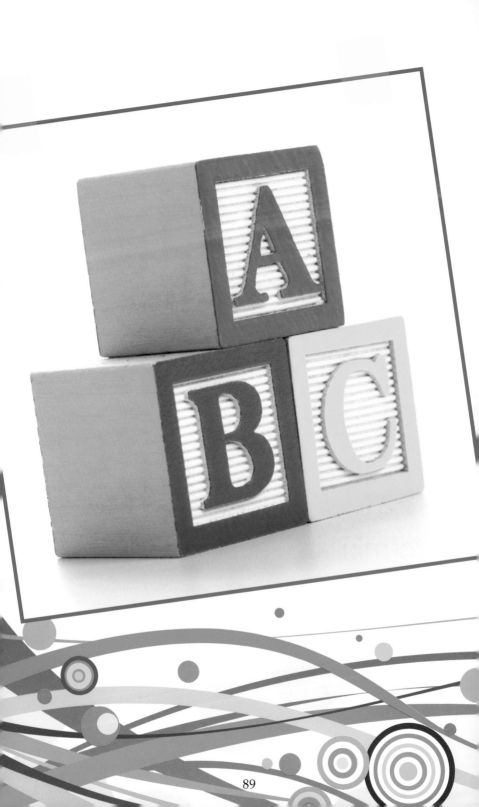

LESS IS MORE

Following the ABC's of my easy steps will insure success in finding the right wig for anyone, regardless of age. Plenty of styling and accessorizing options are available, for everything from an elegant more mature image to more fanciful youthful looks.

In finding just the right hair replacement for the younger set, the first step is identifying the hairstyle she will be accustomed to. This will help her to feel more comfortable with the process.

A current photo of the style, length, and color of the child's hair will be helpful to professionals in determining where to start.

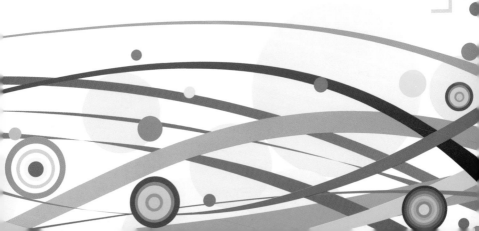

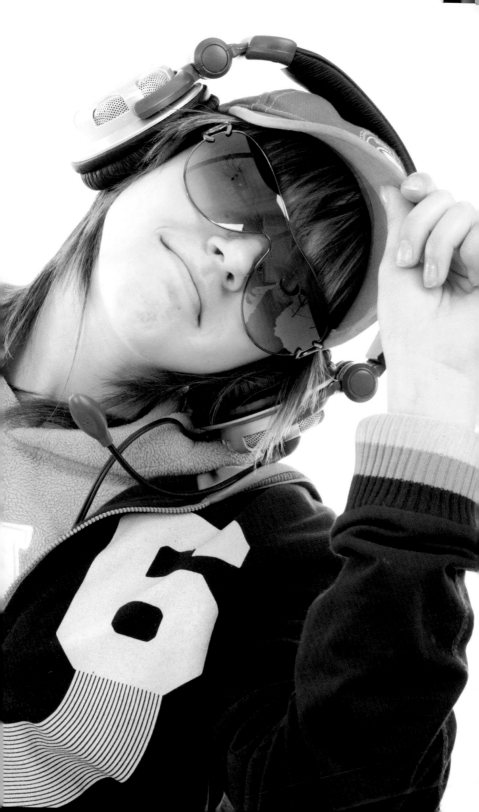

Curl pattern, texture, and color should be matched to what the youngster's natural look.

Fitting a wig for a young person starts with a smaller size cap.

Also, the cap should have considerably less hair than is used in an adult wig.

Almost always these smaller caps will need precise individualized sizing in order to fit them comfortably yet securely. Today's specially designed children's wigs are fully adjustable and provide strategically placed tape pads. Less is more for children's styles.

The use of two-way toupee tape gives much-needed added security for a child's garden of youthful activities.

Once their hair replacement has been selected and fitted, additional personalizing such as added highlights or special styling is always an option. For longer styles natural hair can offer a particularly soft and lifelike look and feel, although many find the amazing tone on tone synthetic color blends of today are just right for younger kids.

One particularly cute yet easy styling idea is to make simple braids with colorful elastic bands arranged to take fullness away from the face. Leave small wisps

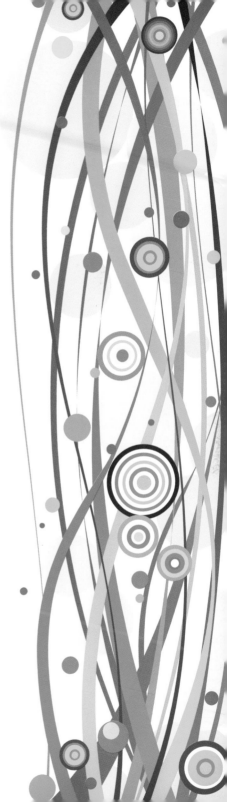

personalizing techniques

open up a *whole*

world of

individuality.

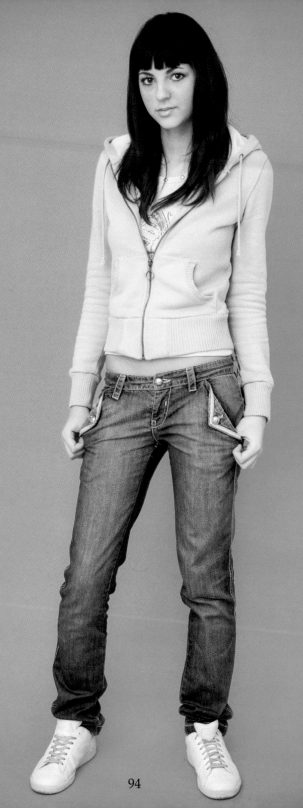

of hair layered around the face to hide the line of the wig. Barrettes, small bows, and petite butterfly clips as well as headbands can add just the right girlish touch.

She can go all out with satin or velvet bows or headbands for special occasions.

Baseball hats and bandannas offer protection from wind and sun for playtime outdoors. Creatively interchanging these fun little options daily will help her feel more comfortable and playful again at a time when life can become "serious." And this advice works at any age, come to think of it.

For her personal time, we recommend sleep caps, turbans, and bandannas. These provide comfort and warmth, and are absorbent in case of night sweats. Colorful head wraps are another alternative cover-up.

Bangs and partial hairpieces work well under hats and caps.

With a child's strenuous activities, daily brushing and fluffing are neccesary to keep their hairpiece looking fresh and natural. All wigs require shampooing after two weeks of daily wear, however some youngsters are much more active and this may call for more

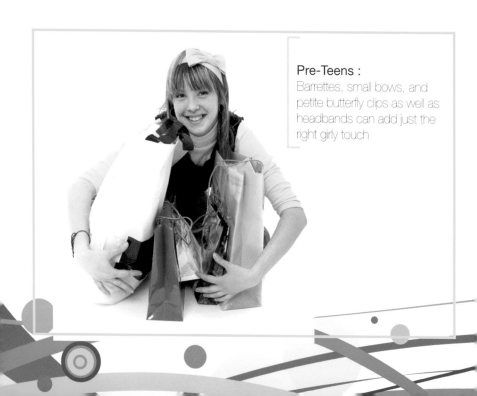

Pre-Teens :
Barrettes, small bows, and petite butterfly clips as well as headbands can add just the right girly touch

frequent attention. It is a practical idea for kids and teenagers to have a backup wig, especially for playtime activities. Alternating will keep things fresher longer.

Teenagers will naturally be more involved with styling and personalizing to express their individuality.

Today's youth culture incorporates many innovative and decorative ideas which can be adapted to their hair replacement. There are extreme "edgy" cuts and colorings patterned after their favorite rock stars and fashion models.

The point here is to allow a feeling of continuity, so their unique self-image is not compromised. The wonderful thing about wigs today is that there are more options than ever before, and personalizing techniques open up a whole world of individuality.

Whether in kindergarten or high school, your child can continue with their plans and activities with ease and practicality. All it takes is a listening ear from the grownups involved and a little ingenuity. This is where all of the ABC's pay off for everyone.

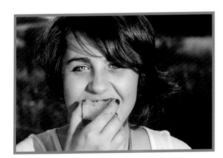

Teenagers :
There are extreme "edgy" cuts and colorings patterned after their favorite rock stars.

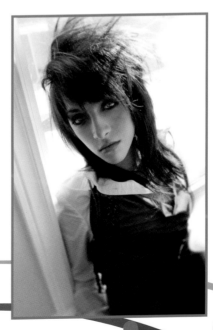

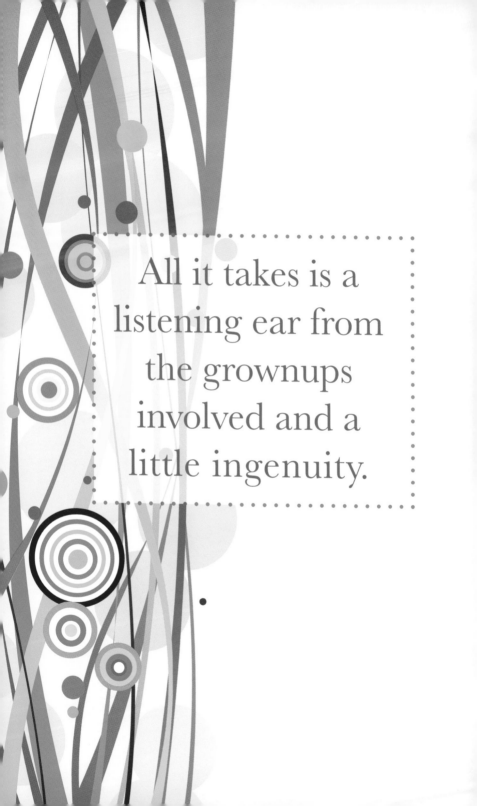

All it takes is a
listening ear from
the grownups
involved and a
little ingenuity.

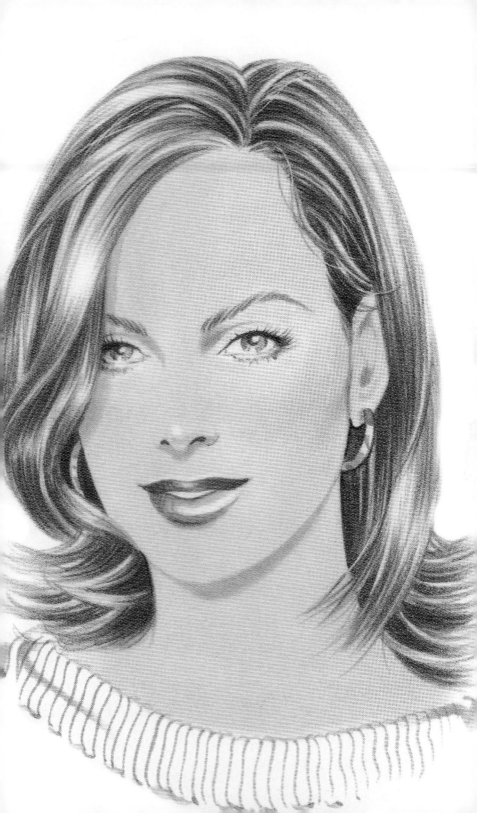

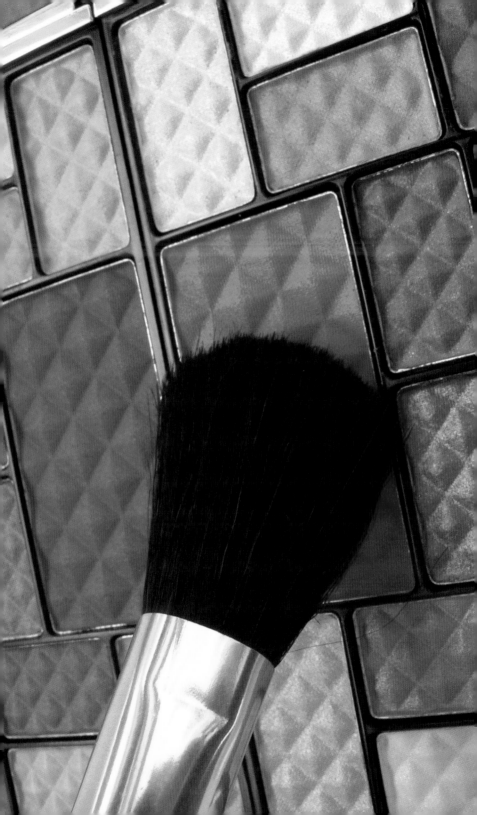

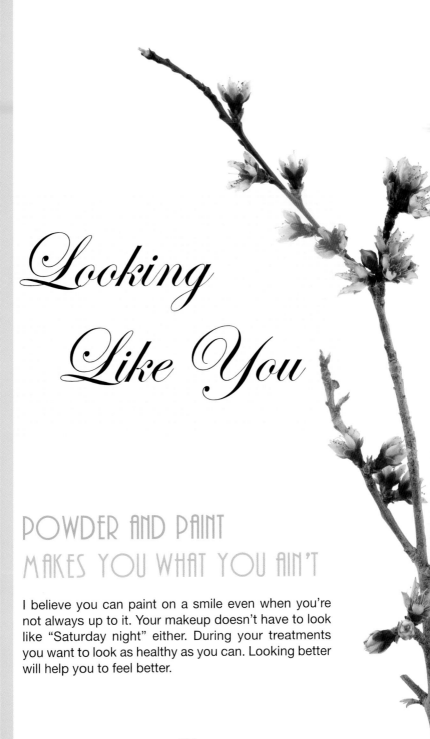

Looking Like You

POWDER AND PAINT
MAKES YOU WHAT YOU AIN'T

I believe you can paint on a smile even when you're not always up to it. Your makeup doesn't have to look like "Saturday night" either. During your treatments you want to look as healthy as you can. Looking better will help you to feel better.

Moisturize your entire body, your face, and your scalp. You might

try a moisturizing foundation

which can help create a healthful glow.

Even if you never wear makeup, you will find it helpful now. Your medication may affect skin tone, often producing a yellow cast. Most makeup lines offer toners called "color correctors," in a variety of colors. Each has its own value. Green cuts red tones. Gold works on ruddy tones. Lavender gives a pinker cast to yellow or olive tones. Lavender or violet is the most useful color in correcting the slightly ash or yellow effect you may experience. These are available in liquids or powders. I recommend the powder form, loose or pressed. Apply lightly, as you would use blush.

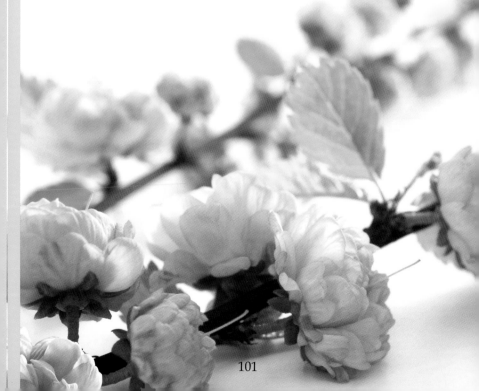

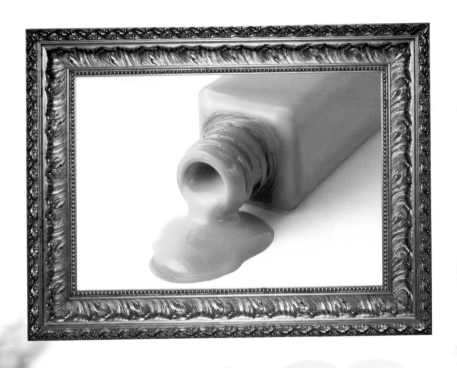

- Green cuts red tones

- Lavender gives a pinker cast to yellow tones.

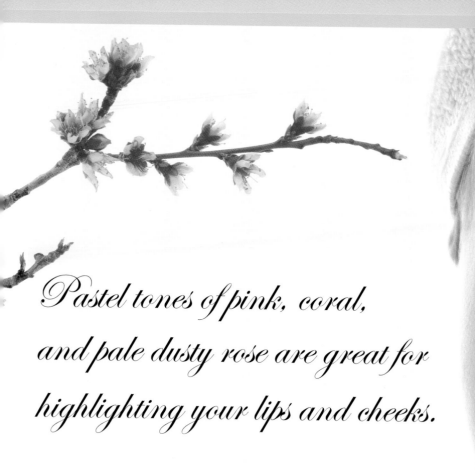

Pastel tones of pink, coral, and pale dusty rose are great for highlighting your lips and cheeks.

For accenting brows, I recommend using a brush-on eyebrow instead of the eyebrow pencil. Eyebrow pencils tend to look drawn and unnatural. Practice drawing the shape of your eyebrows. Most clients tell me they just fill in the missing portions of brows.

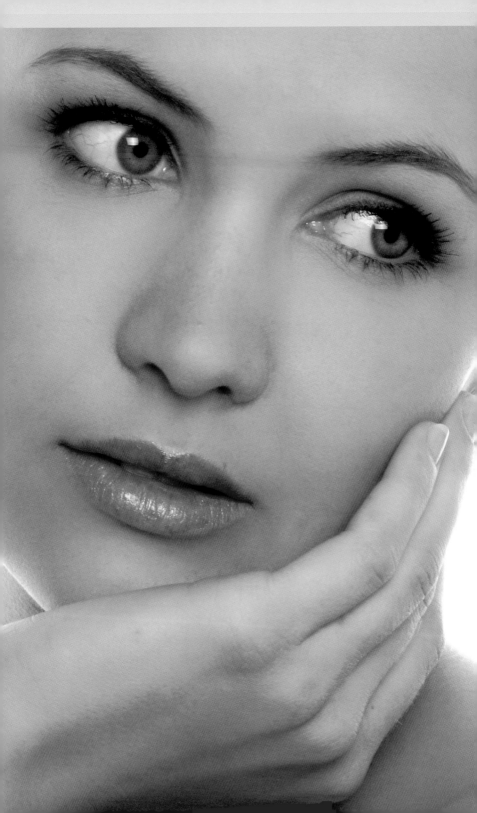

Smudge with a kohl pencil or add individual or false eyelashes to fill in missing lashes. For the most part, only those taking long-term treatments tend to loose all of their brows and lashes.

One of the first things your oncologist will tell you is to avoid people who have colds or flu symptoms. Remember you can "catch a cold" or the flu by sweating from the medication and not covering your head. This can set your whole therapy program back. "Night sweats" are very common with these types of chemotherapy medications. To avoid catching any colds or flu wear a turban or a sleep cap at night. Make sure

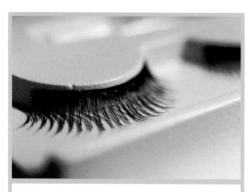

add individual or false eyelashes to **fill** in missing lashes.

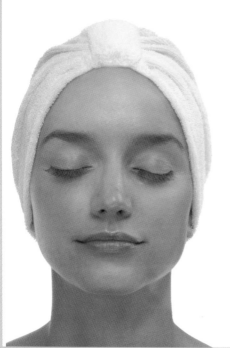

To avoid catching any colds or flu **wear a lightweight cotton sleepcap**

these head coverings are cotton, which is very absorbent. They are very helpful and important for your comfort.

There is a wide range of attractive and practical hair accessories, turbans, headbands, hats and scarves from which to choose.

These allow the freedom to address each individual occasion separately and effectively.

Your look can include a variety of approaches both with and without a wig. With these options you can easily adapt your look to be appropriate anywhere from a wedding to a backyard barbecue.

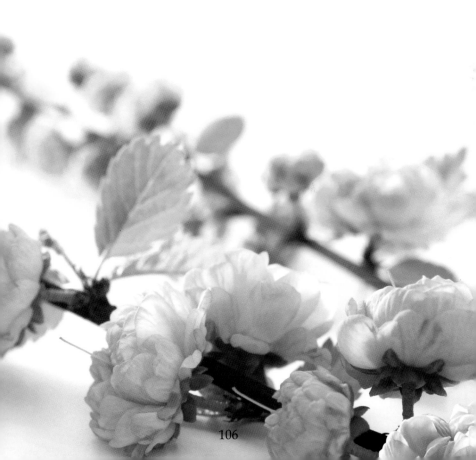

Become comfortable

creating a radiant

healthy glow.

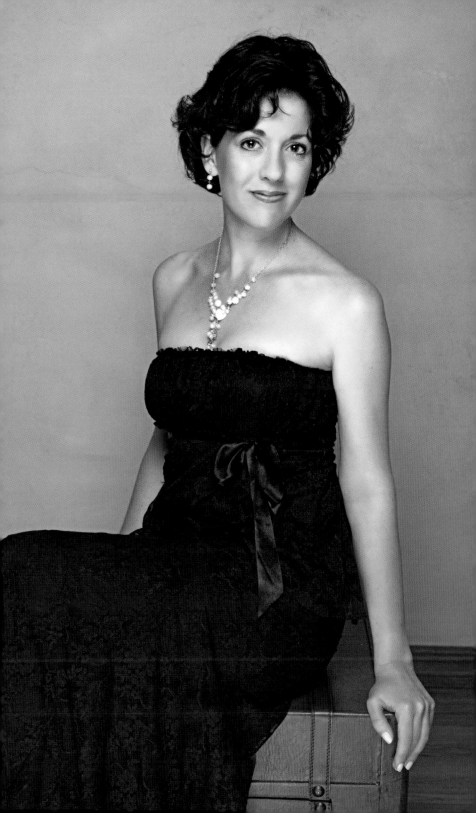

If a special occasion arises when you feel you are not up to it, using one of these simple solution-oriented strategies may enable you to make even just a brief appearance, rather than being a "no-show".

This can be more inspiring to your friends and family than you can ever know.

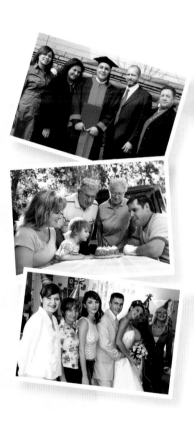

Memorable moments are well worth the effort they may take. Your healthful attitude and appearance will pay off most especially now. Do this for yourself and others.

To avoid unnecessary touch-ups, do your makeup before putting your wig on. You will find it much easier to focus on your features by wearing a turban while applying makeup. Think of this as an everyday routine to both boost your self-confidence and encourage those you love. This benefits everybody, especially you. Become comfortable creating a radiant healthy glow. Your wig and accessories will be the finishing touch. Remember, when you look good, you feel good.

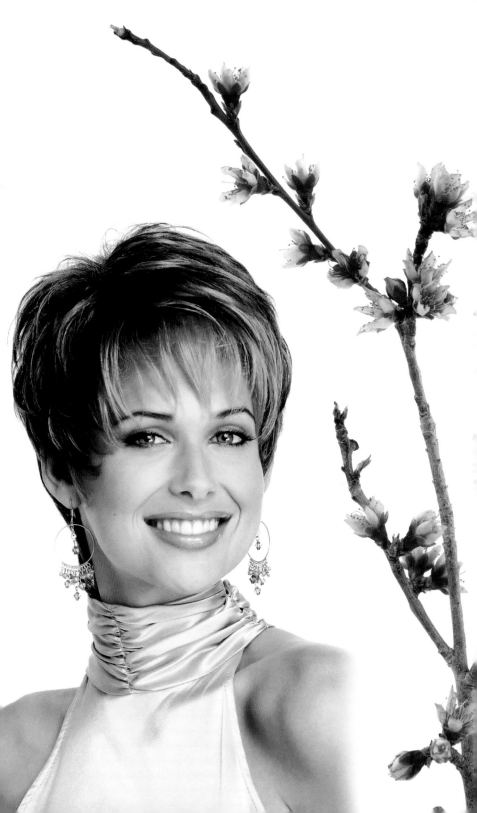

Remember, when
you look good,
you feel good.

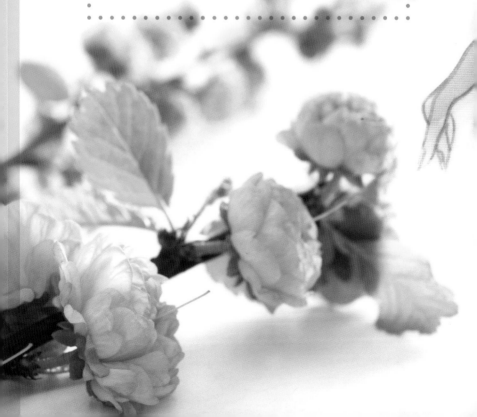

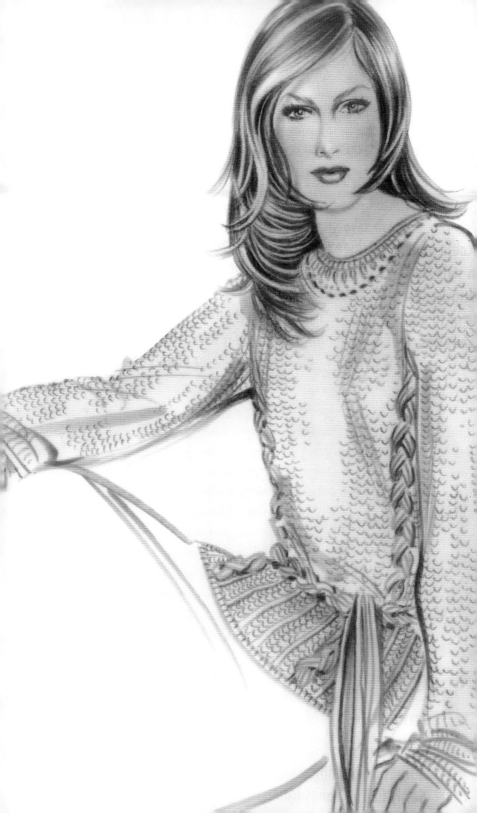

"A light misting of water with a little conditioner mixed in helps with static electricity at any time of year.".

for all Seasons

Looking and feeling great no matter what the thermometer reads can be easily achieved with a plan for all seasons, coordinating hair and makeup with accessories.

Air temperature and humidity will have much the same effect on your hair replacement as it does on your own hair. During hotter weeks, your wig may need washing sooner, after six to eight wearings. It is at these times that many of the fashionable options may come into play to help extend the time between cleanings. In colder climates you may get twelve to fifteen wearings.

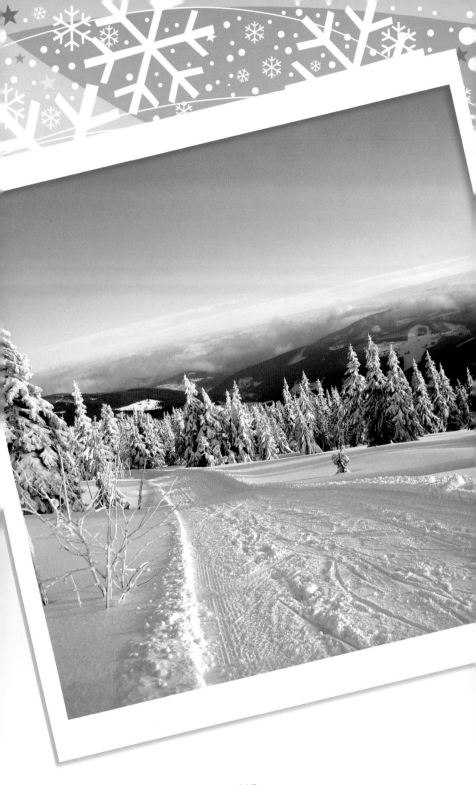

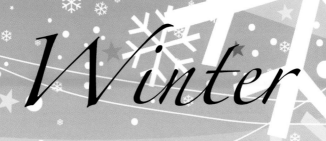

Winter

"There is nothing more *enchanting*
than a brisk walk in a
winter wonderland."

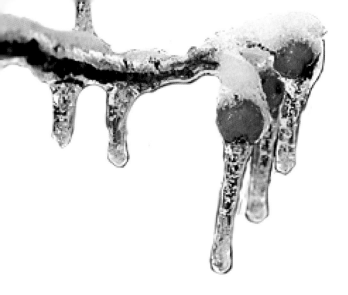

Cozy knit hats with matching scarves and gloves in glorious jewel tones or winter whites will brighten up even the grayest day. Be sure the hat size is large enough to fit over your wig when selecting hats.

A terrific alternative for under thick warm hats or turbans is the "halo of hair." This practical hairpiece consists of a fringe of hair around the circumference of the head with bangs, nape and sides only. You tape it on in place of your full wig. Halos come with velcro attachments that you may use for hats, turbans, and scarves. The halo can be styled and highlighted to look just like your own hair, providing a good-looking workable winter option.

Velour turbans can be teamed with attachable bangs for another cold weather look. Bangs can be styled or thinned, and are particularly well suited for skiwear. Winter turbans and knit hats can also be worn without any hairpiece when the occasion calls for it.

'Tis the season for sparkling hair clips and festive headbands to dress up your hairdo for the holidays. Pull your hair up with a clip, leaving tendrils.

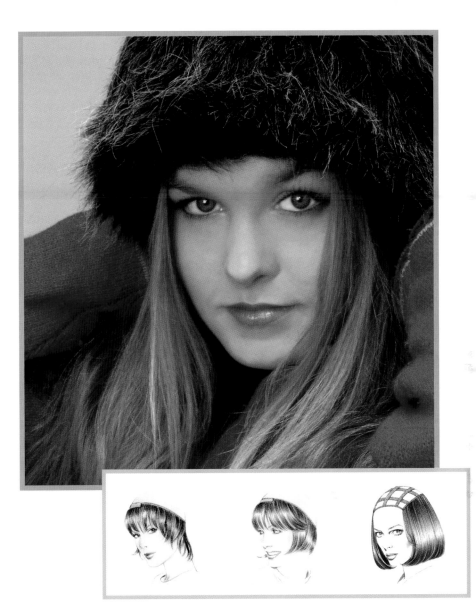

Up: fur hat worn
with "halo of hair."
Right: 3 "halo of
hair" styles.

A luxurious pashmina or cashmere scarf in pale peachy coral, bright deep blue, or a rich garnet red will add the perfect unexpected flash of interesting color right around your face.

Since heated air is drier than normal, use extra moisturizer everywhere.

You might consider using a self-tanning moisturizing bronzer for your complexion. Make sure to always exfoliate before applying self-tanning, and cover your neck, shoulders, and arms for an even glow.

You'll look splendid in that little black dress for holiday dinner parties.

Makeup for winter's paler complexion can be kept clean and simple. Enhance your cheeks with apricot or rose tones. For eyes use neutral taupes and warm pale browns with shimmery gold highlights. Try lipsticks in deep rich sheer raspberries and mauves with a dab of golden gloss. Classic reds on lips and nails look fabulous with black. Evenings start earlier, so your winter look can be subtle yet dressy. Have the happiest of holidays.

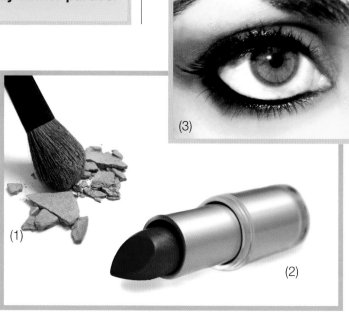

(3)

From left to right:
(1) soft rose blush for cheeks.
(2) classic red for lips.
(3) taupe eye shadows with hints of gold.

(1)

(2)

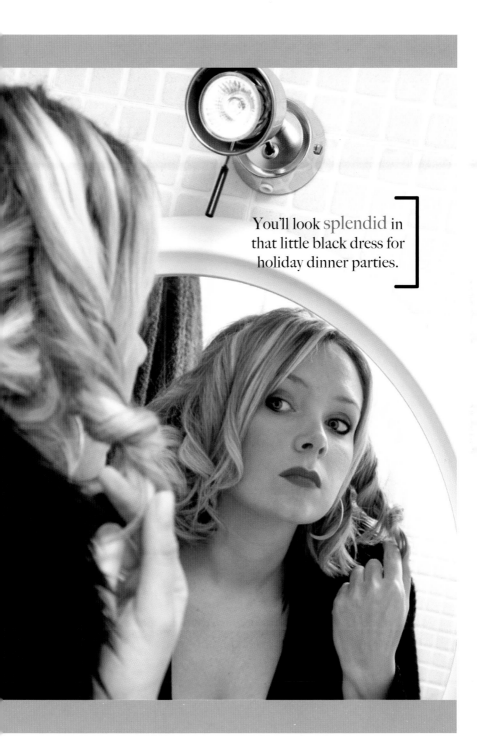

You'll look splendid in that little black dress for holiday dinner parties.

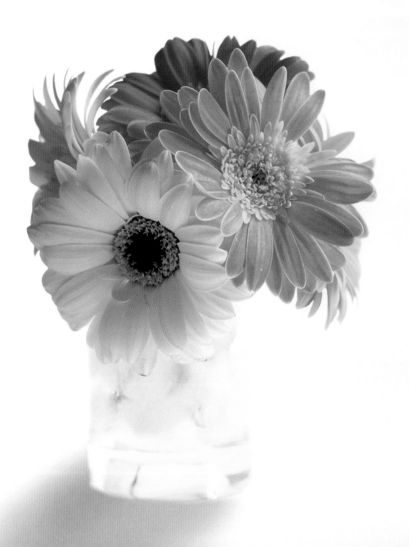

SP

RING

This is nature's time of renewal, when everything from a whole forest to a blade of grass gets a fresh new start. Flowers are in bloom again and skies are blue. It's time to bring in lively floral pastel colors and shake off the heavier, richer hues of winter.

Wear turbans, head wraps, and scarves in *lighter fabrics.*

Perhaps a brooch or pin can bring a lovely seasonal accent. Headbands can come into play to secure your hairpiece on windy days. Think light and breezy in stylizing for spring, taking a decidedly more casual approach. This works for your hairstyling as well as makeup and fashion.

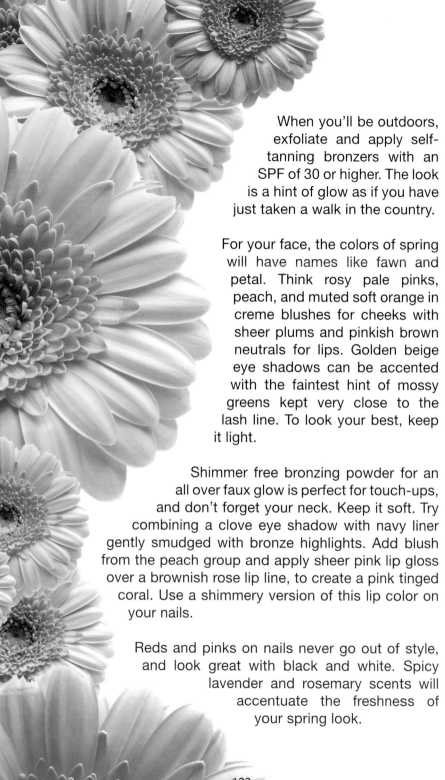

When you'll be outdoors, exfoliate and apply self-tanning bronzers with an SPF of 30 or higher. The look is a hint of glow as if you have just taken a walk in the country.

For your face, the colors of spring will have names like fawn and petal. Think rosy pale pinks, peach, and muted soft orange in creme blushes for cheeks with sheer plums and pinkish brown neutrals for lips. Golden beige eye shadows can be accented with the faintest hint of mossy greens kept very close to the lash line. To look your best, keep it light.

Shimmer free bronzing powder for an all over faux glow is perfect for touch-ups, and don't forget your neck. Keep it soft. Try combining a clove eye shadow with navy liner gently smudged with bronze highlights. Add blush from the peach group and apply sheer pink lip gloss over a brownish rose lip line, to create a pink tinged coral. Use a shimmery version of this lip color on your nails.

Reds and pinks on nails never go out of style, and look great with black and white. Spicy lavender and rosemary scents will accentuate the freshness of your spring look.

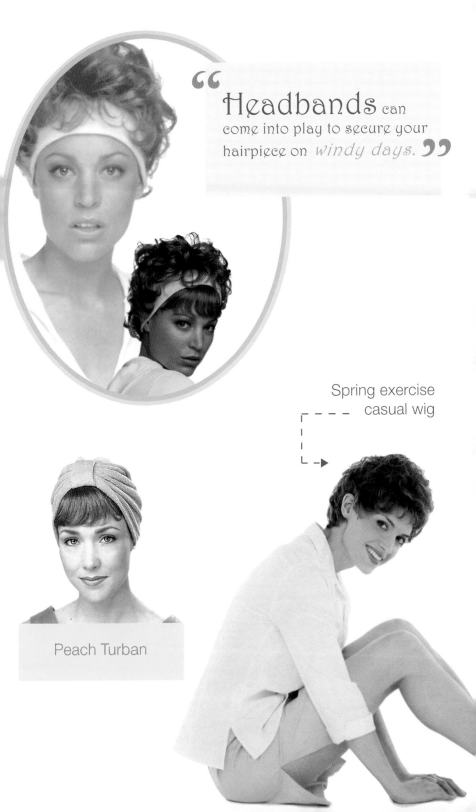

> **Headbands** can come into play to secure your hairpiece on *windy days.*

Spring exercise casual wig

Peach Turban

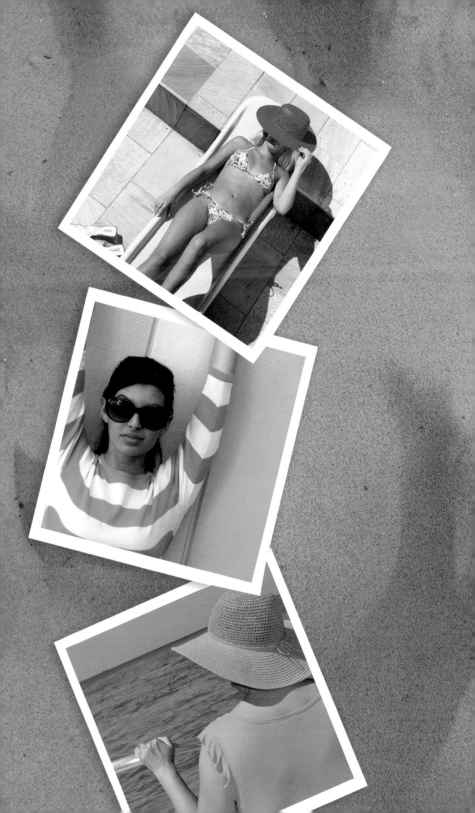

Summer

**In summertime,
the livin' is easy.**

You can enjoy the sun without
soaking it up. You'll have it
"made in the shade" with big
brimmed hats. Keep a visor
in your car.

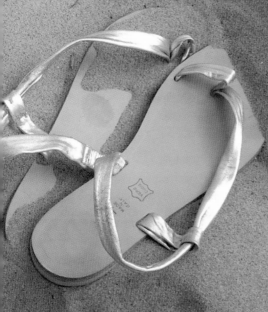

Large sheer scarves double up as a shoulder wrap to shield sensitive shoulders from the sun. Have changes of loose clothing for hot weather, which can be added or shed as needed.

Hoop earrings look great with a summer dress and vanilla bean tan. Use moisturizing bronzers or self-tanning lotion with a stronger SPF 45. You want to look like you have been basking in the sun, not baking in it.

Refresh your complexion with rose water and other soothing botanical mists, which provide aromatherapy as well as much needed moisture. Mist as often as you like. Include your hairpiece. During heat spells it is especially important to sip water constantly. For those who swim, find a swim cap that covers the head and ear area completely. After your swim you might mist the ends of your wig to appear as if you have just towel dried your hair.

> "During heat spells it is especially important to sip water constantly."
>
> "Wake up to chilled fruit to recharge your energy."

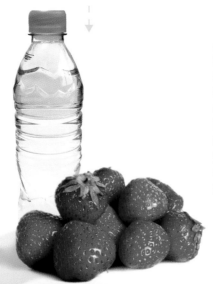

Avoid becoming overtired by taking occasional fifteen-minute naps, with your feet elevated. Cool refrigerated eye pads are very soothing. Wake up to iced herbal or green tea and chilled fresh fruit to recharge your energy. During the longer daylight hours napping really helps stabilize your energy.

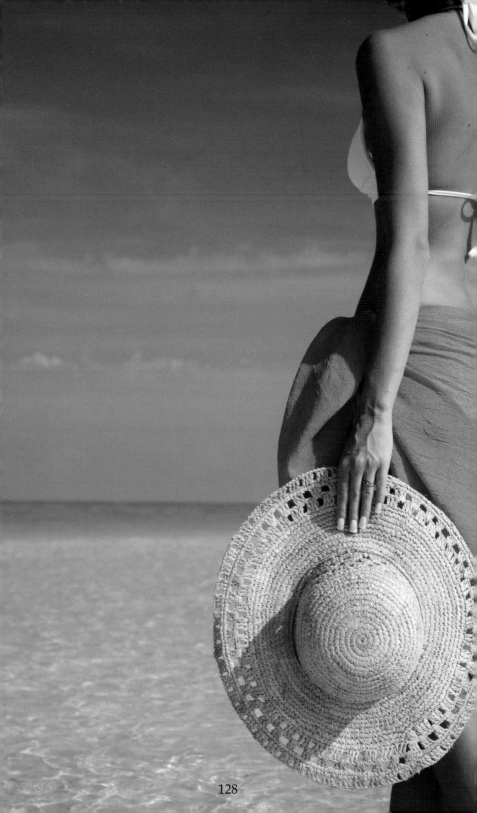

Small barrettes add lift and interest to the sides of your wig. Alternative options become especially relevant for your comfort now. A turban with 3/4 wig is chic with the season's more casual evening wear. Straw boaters or lovely white large brims can be teamed with the halo of hair. A white absorbent cotton turban with optional bangs is a classic staple.

A really clever idea one client shared with me was to install loops on the inside rim of your sun hat. You thread a long lightweight scarf through the loop to act as a strap. It's so versatile to be able to mix and match any scarf. For times when you don't wish to wear any hairpiece, you can tie a scarf as a head wrap under the sun hat, using the loops to secure it.

Treat yourself to a pedicure. Champagne nail polish with a hint of shimmer won't compete with your bronzed summer face. Nails are best kept shorter and neutral, in metallic shades.

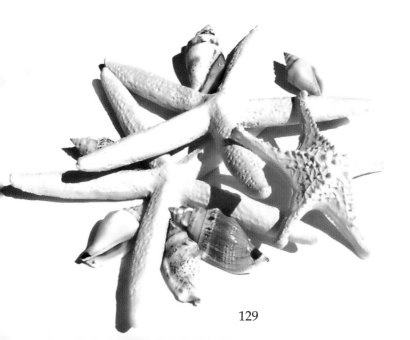

Your makeup strategy is "barely there." Use a light hand on mascara and liner, they can run in the heat. Darker complexions can wear darker reddish brown on lips, and lighter complexions do better with sheer stains in bright corals and pinks. You can lighten up any lip color with a pale lip pencil drawn just inside the lip line, over the lipstick. It works to make thin lips look fuller also. Add a dab of gold gloss. This clean sparkling look will take you everywhere from a picnic to the country club.

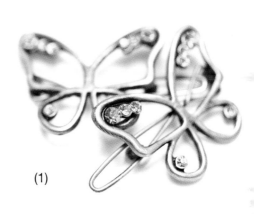

(1)

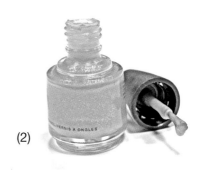

(2)

(3)

From top to bottom:
(1) barrettes
(2) champagne
nail polish
(3) treat yourself to
a pedicure...

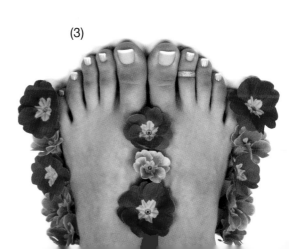

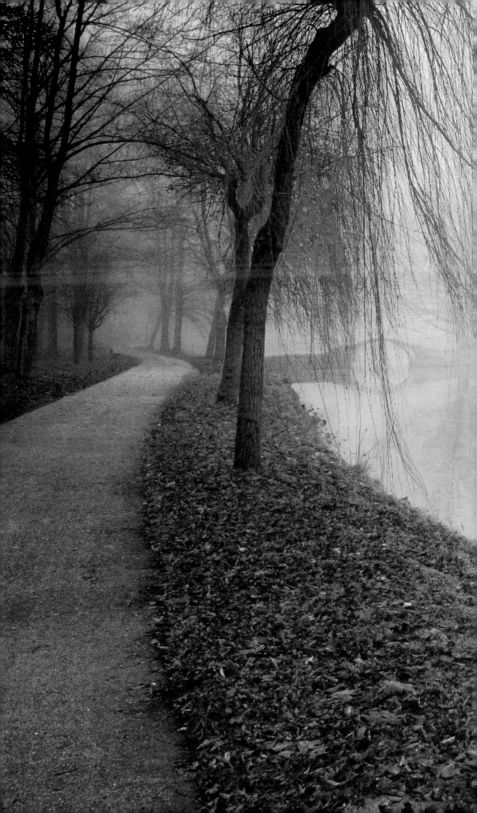

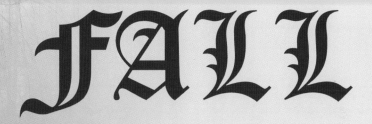

FALL

As Indian summer fades to autumn, renew your spirits with a picnic with friends.

Take longer walks through the changing foliage taking full advantage of the crisper air.

Stretch time spent outdoors in preparation for the shorter days to come. Take in a sunset then dine later under the harvest moon.

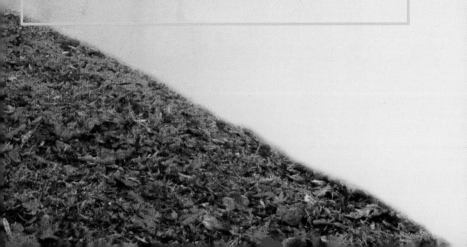

It's time for the transition from summer's casualness to a more structured approach to fashion. Your hairstyle can reflect this. Consider having your wig restyled for a sleeker look to better enhance tailored jackets, vests, and the smaller sunglasses and hats of the season. It may be refreshing to trim and refine the look just a touch. Change is in the air.

Autumn makeup colors are earthy and natural. Pale neutral eyes combine with brick red creme formulas on lips with a touch of shine. Sweep charcoal or rich brown shadow across the eyelid to the outer corner to form a soft point.

down: sleeker hair with smaller sunglasses

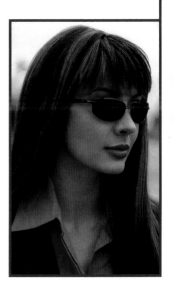

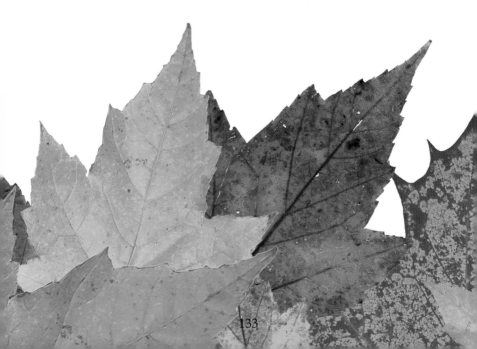

**down: earthy, natural shades of makeup.
ethnic golden brown.
down-right: brown shadow with touch of shine**

Think smoky, and blend softly. Add opal shimmer highlights. Pale brownish rose blush will give a subtle contrast to brighter richer cranberry or plum in sheer lip stains. The look is fresh, warm, and classic.

With more makeup, think less nail polish. Very neutral browns, shiny nudes, or pale rose are softly vibrant. Shorter nails work best for many at this busy time of year.

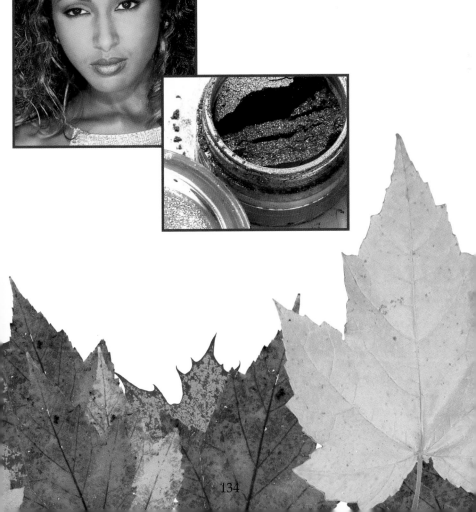

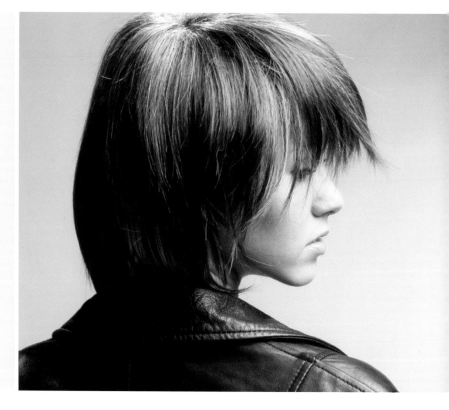

Wear and Care

Throughout each chapter I have sprinkled advice and useful tips. Now we'll put all the basics you need together for easy reference.

Observe how people relate to their hair. Notice how some fling it around to make a point, or flip their bangs off their face. Others gesture at the nape of the neck absentmindedly. That is how naturally and comfortably you want to relate to your wig.

Run your fingers softly through your hair. Lightly fluff and finger style your wig just like you do with your own hair. Touch your hair in expressive gestures. This makes all the difference in the natural appearance of your hair replacement, and your comfort in wearing it. You will find that by consciously making this effort in the beginning, it will soon come naturally. Feel relaxed about touching your hair and moving your head freely, nodding, gesturing, feeling the breeze, Looking Like You...

You'll want to maintain the crisp look of your personalized and freshly styled new wig. Today's wigs are very easy to clean with cold water and unscented shampoos.

Even if your wig still looks good on the outside, oils and perspiration collect inside the cap, requiring regular cleaning. However, shampooing a wig more than once every two weeks will eventually dehydrate the fibers, making your wig look dry and unnatural.

There may be the occasional exception to this rule when an activity has resulted in the need for additional cleaning, but remember that this is not your hair and you don't need to shampoo it every day.

Gentle but thorough brushing will refresh and rejuvenate the style between wearings. For straighter styles use a wire brush. Use only a wig-pick or vent brush on curly styles to keep the curls intact, fluffing lightly. Avoid using standard hair brushes on any hairpiece, as these can create excessive tension, over-stressing the hair with abrasive strokes.

Think in reverse when brushing any wig. Start from the ends and work gradually toward the root area, directly opposite as you would with your own hair. When using a wire pick also work the curls from the ends to the root area.

A light misting with water with a little conditioner mixed in will rejuvenate any style. For touch-ups between washings, lightly mousse, hand scrunch and pick the style into curls. For straight styles mousse and brush lightly.

You might also use electric or steam molecular rollers to reinforce the curl pattern. Remember that very hot styling tools such as curling irons will damage synthetic fibers. However these irons can be very useful for pieces made with human hair. Keeping your hairpiece fresh and clean will add to its beauty and longevity.

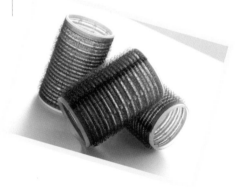

Cleaning
Synthetic Wigs

- After two weeks of wear your wig should be cleaned with cold water and unscented shampoo. During warmer weather this may be neccesary more often.

- Washing your synthetic wig in hot water will alter the original curl pattern or damage the synthetic fiber.

- Make sure to put shampoo into the cold water and not directly on the wig.

- Dip your hairpiece up and down in the water three or four times, then rinse thoroughly. Rinse again. Towel blot then shake vigorously.

- Brush lightly and air dry on a wig stand or hang to dry.

- Never dry a wig on a flat surface, this may crush the curl.

- When completely dry simply brush and restyle.

- A folding wig stand is a useful alternative to a styrofoam wig head. You can carry one in your kit, and keep one on your dressing table. The advantage of these forms is that the ventilation allows the inside of the cap to air out and dry.

- Styrofoam wig heads can be too large, and may stretch your wig, affecting the fit. Wigs tend to lose their elasticity on foam heads. It is important not to use any head or form that will loosen the fit once your wig has been sized.

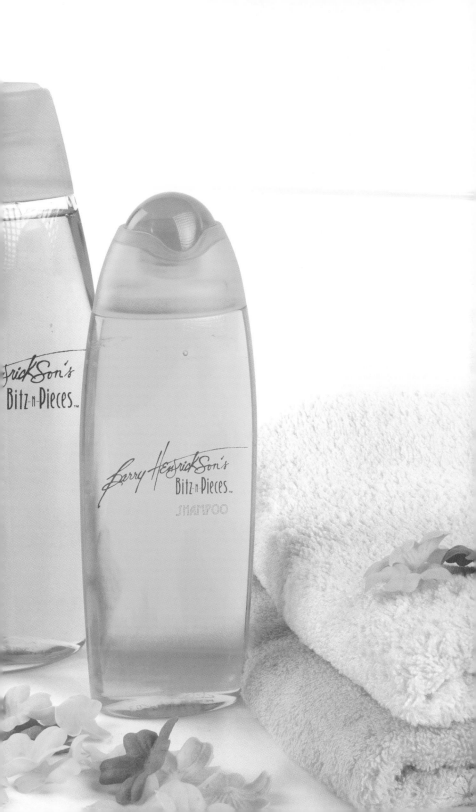

Cleaning Tips
for Natural Hair

There are special considerations for washing and styling real hair wigs. Today's ready to wear styles made with human hair may be washed in cold or lukewarm water just the same as with synthetics. The main difference is how you condition and restyle human hair or human hair blended with synthetic.

After rinsing all shampoo out of the hairpiece, apply the conditioner treatment directly on the damp hair, starting at the end of the hair shaft and working towards the root area. After leaving the conditioner on the hair for 10 to 15 minutes, rinse thoroughly and restyle. Keep conditioner off the root area of hand-knotted wigs as it will eventually loosen the hair and cause the hair to thin and fall out.

It is best to let the piece air-dry before styling. This way you are styling freshly cleaned hair that is conditioned and silky.

Slip the wig onto a canvas wig head, (also called a "block"), using T-pins to hold the wig in place. The wig head fits onto a wig clamp which gives you complete control of your working angle, allowing you to

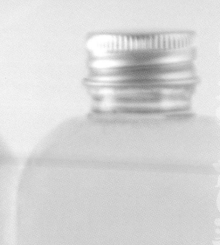

easily stylize your wig using a wet set, electric rollers, blowers or a curling iron.

Remember that synthetic fiber is less heat resistant than human hair, so it's best not to use a curling iron on any synthetic, even if it is blended with human hair.

A custom wig should be blocked on a canvas wig head your own size for washing and restyling. This will prevent your cap from stretching out of shape or the hair from reversing to the inside of the cap. When working on hairpieces with lace front hairlines you must be extra careful not to rip or tear the delicate lace netting. Pin a ribbon along the hairline to secure it in place and protect from stretching, ripping and fraying while styling. Carefully dab special cleaning solvent as neccesary to remove the dried glue.

A wig dry cleaning solution may be used in place of shampoo and water to preserve the color and curl, and avoid excess tangling.

By using these methods you'll get the best looking results, just like the professionals.

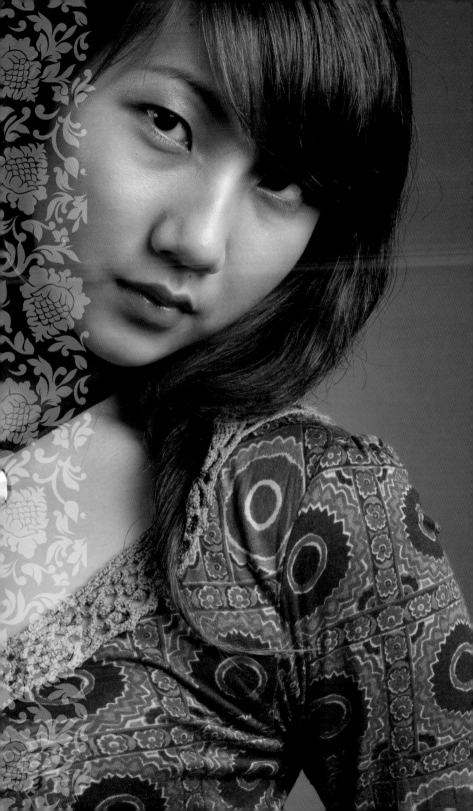

Styling Tips

Here are some clear and simple styling tips to easily retouch and refresh your wig whenever needed:

Shake and brush out your wig before each wearing.

For short styles lightly mist with water then gently arrange into the style.

Try today's regular hair products such as styling mousse or gels, as needed. Be careful not to over-do it.

For human hair or blends use your regular hair shampoo and add conditioner for normal to dry hair.

Adjustable tabs on the inside of the wig assure a good fit. Some use velcro tabs or adjustable eye hooks, or slides.

Both natural and synthetic hair can be set with steam or electric rollers for a quick fix, or a last-minute touch-up.

Excessive heat from curling irons damages synthetic fiber, so curling irons should be avoided. Curling irons should be used for human hair only.

For those experienced with curling irons, you may use steam curling irons only on a lower setting to retouch or reinforce the curl pattern of a synthetic.

Never lay your wig down on a flat surface overnight. It will lose its shape and the curl pattern will flatten.

When setting your wig with rollers you will need to place it on a canvas wig block. These blocks are available in different sizes. Use T-pins to secure the wig before you start setting.

Lace front and custom wigs must always be carefully blocked with T-pins on a canvas wig block to maintain their delicate shape.

For a human hair wig, allowing your set to air dry will result in a firmer set, allowing the curl to hold longer.

When your hair is not becoming to you, it's time for you to be coming to us.

Many wig salons offer a cleaning service. We have found that clients may not want to deal with cleaning wigs during their treatments.

If you are unable to get to the salon, family or friends are happy to deliver and pick up your wigs. You might ask if you can mail it to the salon to be serviced. Your stylist should be familiar with your style and return it to you looking fresh and clean. If you can't get the wig to the salon regularly, at least have it done professionally every so often, perhaps every third shampoo. This gives both you and your wig a great perk.

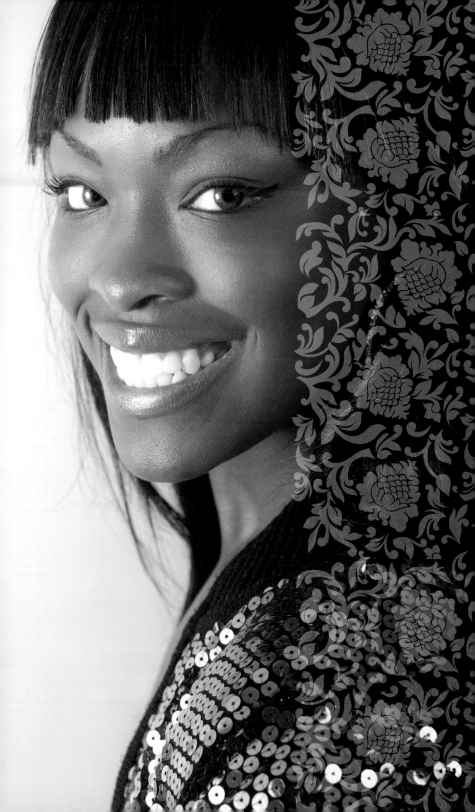

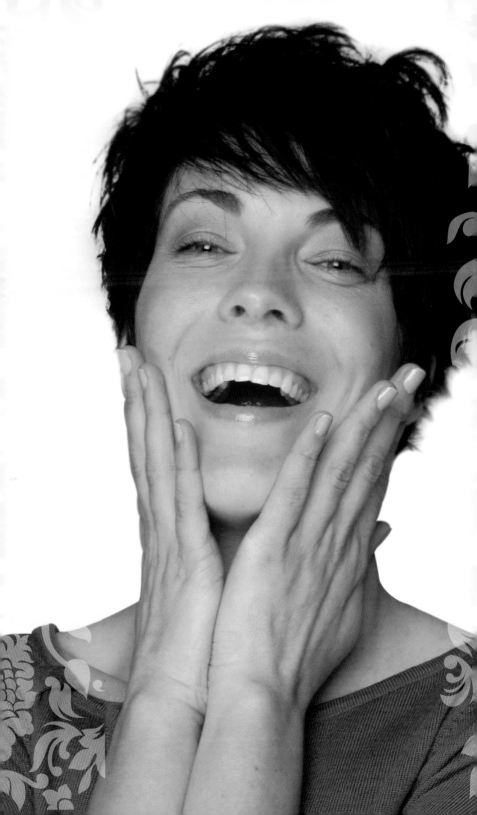

Consider this a Day of Beauty, time just for you to refurbish your hairpiece's style and have it freshly applied and fluffed. You will enjoy this treat. You may wish to visit a nail salon for a manicure and pedicure. You can also have a soothing massage and facial. This can really help you to look good, and as a result, feel better.

Some get through the hair loss, treatments, and then regrowth with only one wig. That's a lot to ask of one wig. If this is the case, it's advisable to get a new wig when your hair starts growing back. The same style, but a fresh one, will not only feel better, but this will allow room for the new hair that is growing in. This will also give you a fresh outlook.

In most cases, your hair will grow back just the same as it was. Sometimes, however, it can grow back in a different color or texture.

Take the time to assemble your "just in case" kit. Keep it simple and keep it with you wherever you go. Taking careful care of yourself and your hairpieces will help you to relax and concentrate on enjoying life.

You can never hear this too many times: when you look good, you feel good.

It's a simple truth. It is so reassuring and comforting to your family and friends when you flash that radiant smile at them, Looking Like You...

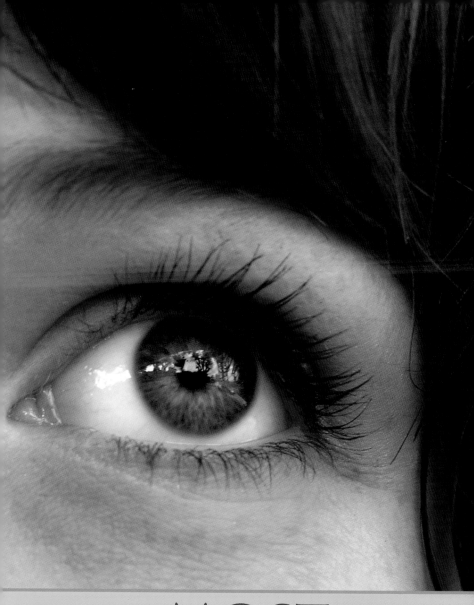

MOST
FREQUENTLY
ASKED

Q | What is the first thing I need to know about choosing my wig?

A *Consider all types of wigs available. Choose from synthetics, blends, or natural hair wigs. Synthetics are ready-to-wear and easy to care for. Blends contain synthetic fiber mixed with human hair, and require more styling. Natural hair and custom wigs require proper washing and should be restyled by a salon every so often.*

Q | What is the difference between ready-to-wear and custom?

A *Ready to wear wigs are machine made or a combination of machine and handmade. Custom wigs start wtih a handmade cap, then each hair is hand-knotted in a process called ventilating, (which is a lot like crocheting).*

Q | How can I match my own texture and color?

A *Today's colors are achieved by blending at least three different shades of the same color tone on tone, creating highlights. Your favorite blond, brunette, or reds are available. In some cases, a closer match to your color tone can be achieved by coloring with a temporary color rinse.*

Q | How can I make my wig fit comfortably?

A *Adjustable tabs on the inside of the wig assure a good fit. Some use velcro tabs or adjustable eye hooks. If the wig feels too large you may size it. I always recommend professional help. First start with the depth of the cap. Sizing is accomplished by removing a few wefts, (rows of hair), in the crown area or nape area. Carefully cut between the rows of hair then sew the sections back together. Never remove more than three wefts in any one section. The circumference is made tighter by sewing a tuck on the elastic in the area behind the ear. The proper fit is snug but not too tight, guaranteeing you'll look good and feel good.*

Q | How can I make my wig look more natural?

A *Ready to wear styles often are too heavy around your face. Have your wig styled. Simply thinning the hairline frames your face, making all the difference in appearance. Have a professional help you with this all-important procedure. Never over-thin your wig. If you change the volume too much, you can lose the whole look of the style. For a more natural look keep your style the most flattering length and thickness for your facial shape. You can always cut it, but remember it won't grow back.*

Q | When and how do I clean my wig?

A *After two weeks of wear your wig should be cleaned with cold water and unscented shampoo. Washing your wig in hot water will alter the original curl pattern and damage the fiber. Make sure to put shampoo into the water and not directly on the wig. Dip it up and down in the suds three or four times, then rinse thoroughly. Rinse again. Towel blot then shake vigorously. Brush lightly and air dry on a wig stand or hang to dry. Styrofoam forms tend to stretch-out the cap. Never dry a wig flat; this may crush the curl. When it's completely dry you may brush and restyle.*

Q | How can I refresh my wig between wearings?

A *Shake and brush out your wig before each wearing. It will retain its natural look when it is soft and fresh. For short styles lightly mist with water then gently arrange into the style. Try using hair products such as styling mousse or gels. This will reduce volume for a younger and more natural look.*

> **Q** How do I revive the curl?

Synthetic hair can be set with steam or electric rollers. Excessive heat from curling irons damage the fiber so curling irons should be avoided. With human hair you may use curling irons, wet roller settings, electric rollers, and blow dryers. For the best results, occasionally have your wig professionally restyled.

> **Q** How do I order a wig if I'm bedridden in the hospital or at home?

Measure the circumference of your head, and then the distance from the hairline to the nape of the neck to determine your wig size. When providing this information to the wig salon, be sure to include a sample of your hair for color and texture, and a photo of yourself in the hairstyle you would like to match. The stylist can take it from there. Your hospital attendant may be able to refer you to someone who provides this service.

> **Q** How should I approach my health insurance for reimbursement?

Ask your oncologist for a prescription for your wig. Your doctor will call it a Medical Hair Prosthetic or a durable medical equipment. When you speak to your health provider about coverage on wigs, always refer to it as a "Medical Hair Prosthetic or a Durable Medical Equipment." Please note that wigs are considered a cosmetic cover-up, and are not covered by insurance. Therefore, make sure your receipt states that it is a Medical Hair Prosthetic purchase or a Durable Medical Equipment. Make copies of both the prescription and the store receipts for your records. Often they get lost and you want to able to present them to your insurance company, if asked.

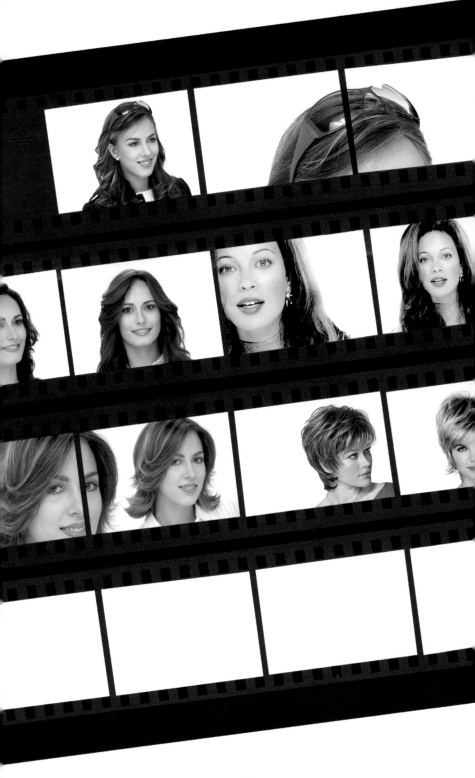

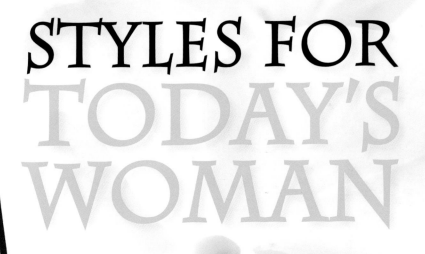

STYLES FOR TODAY'S WOMAN

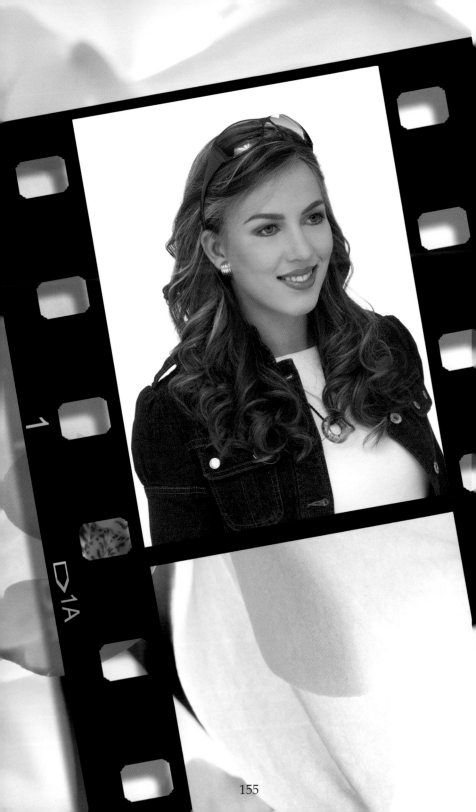

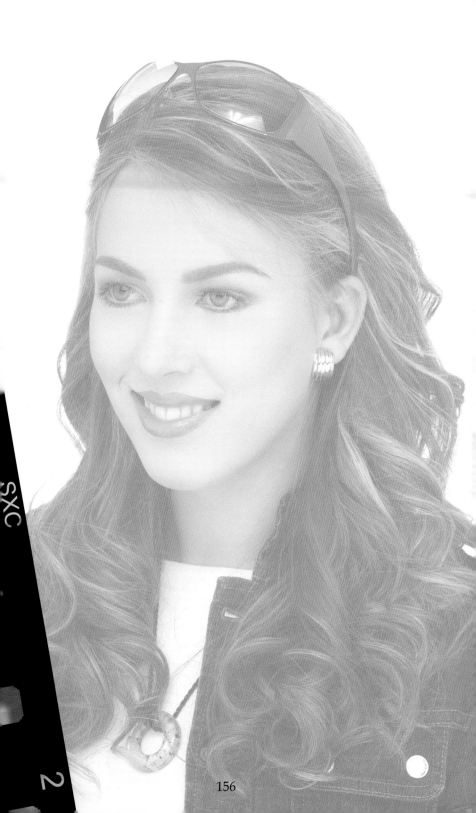

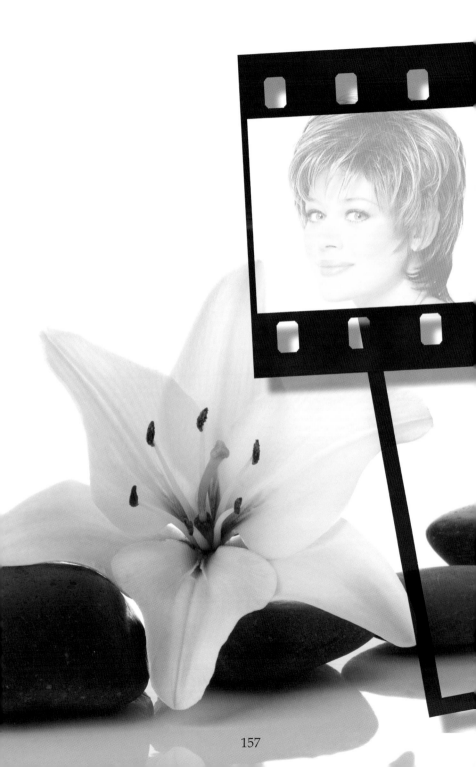

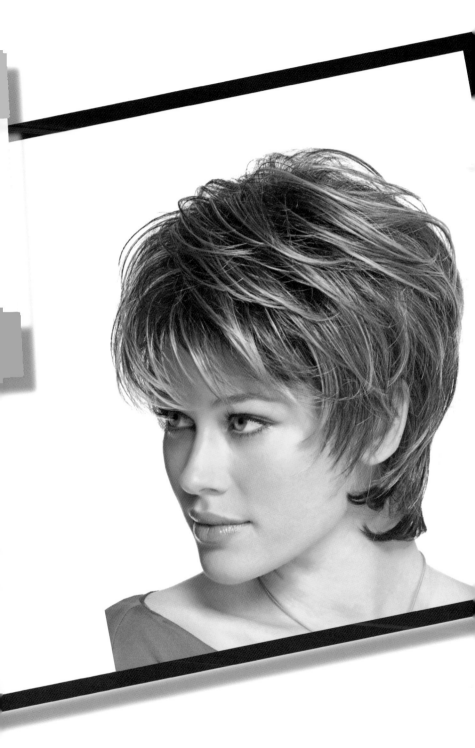

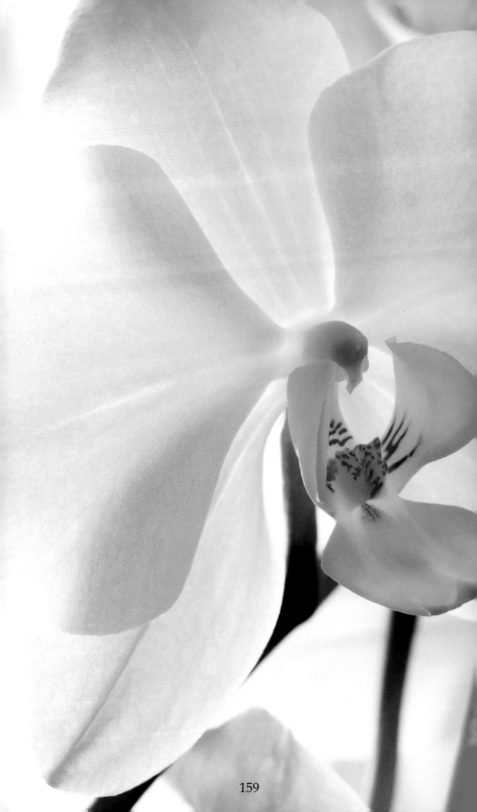

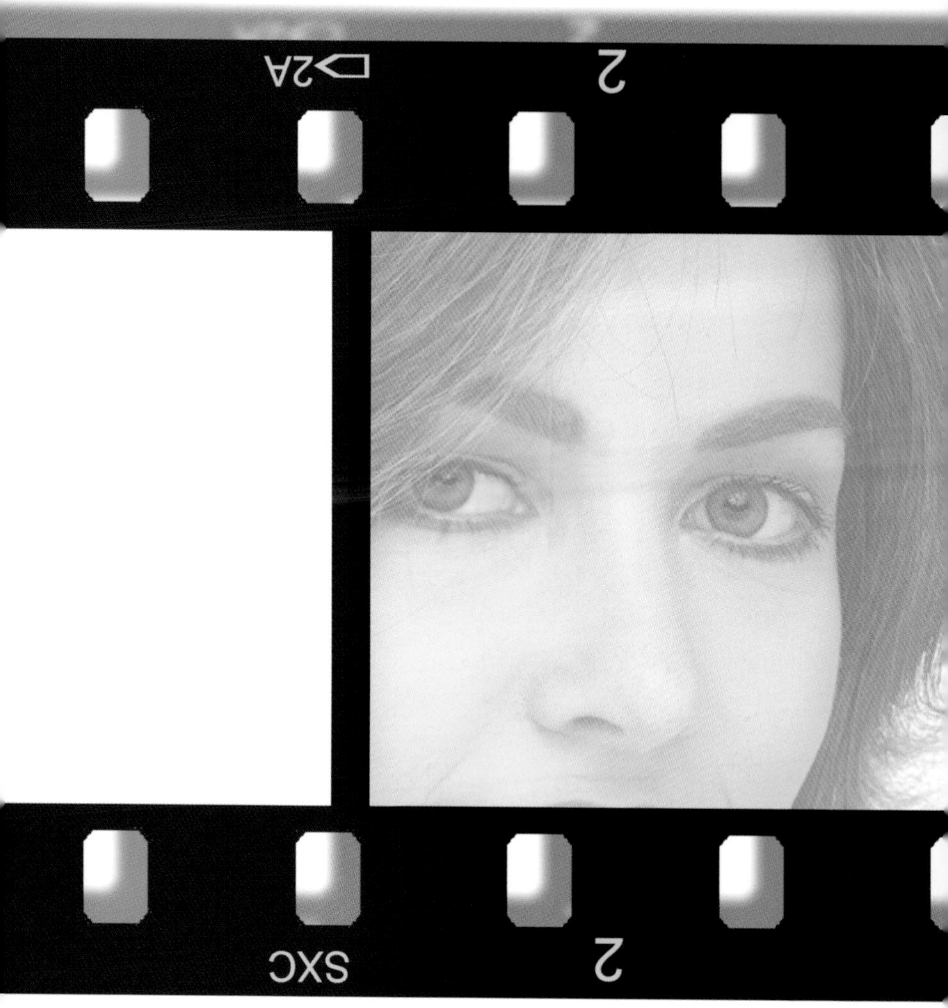
2A
2
SXC
2

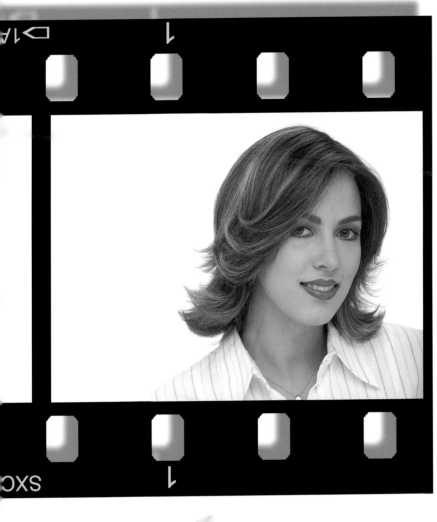

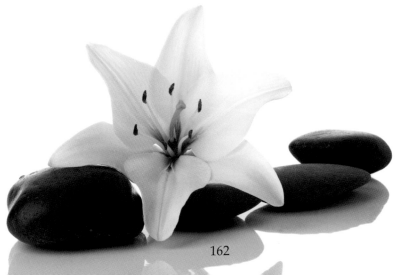

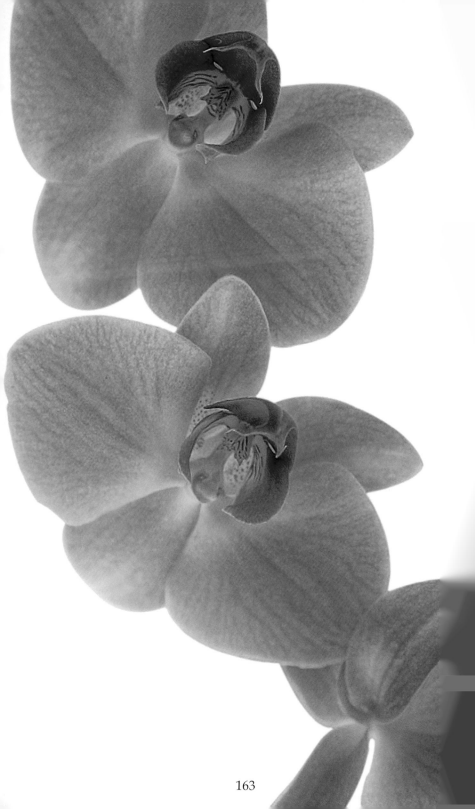

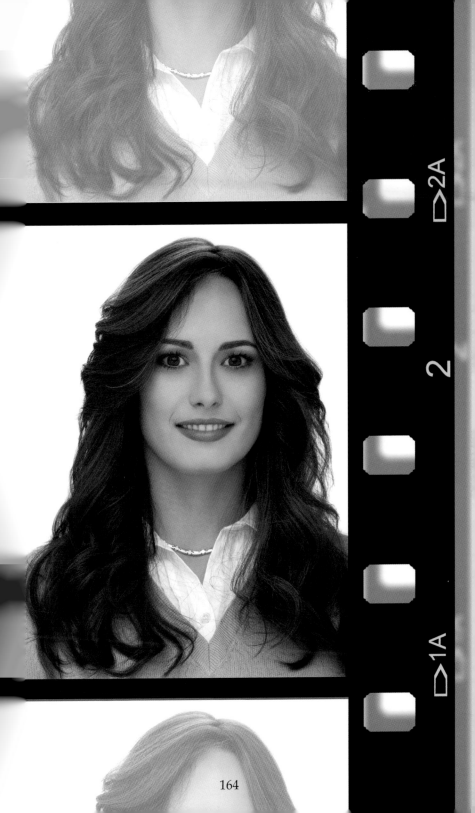

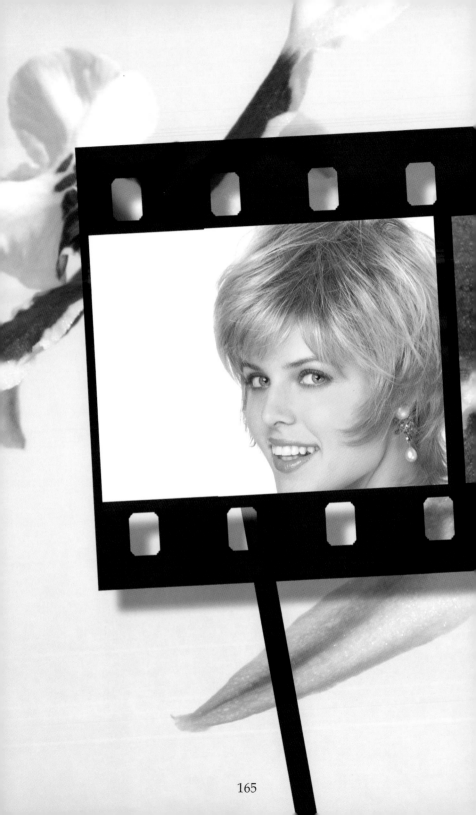

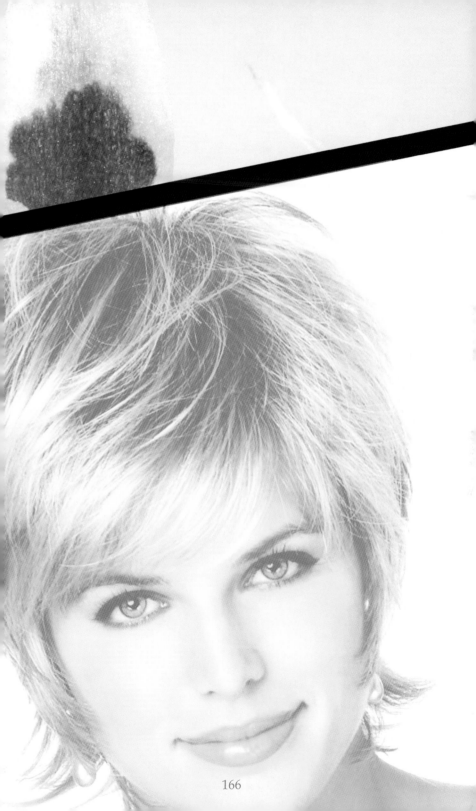

166

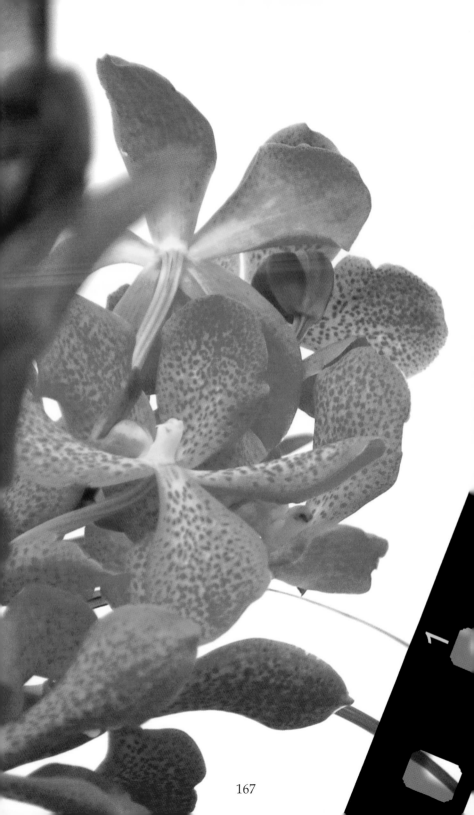

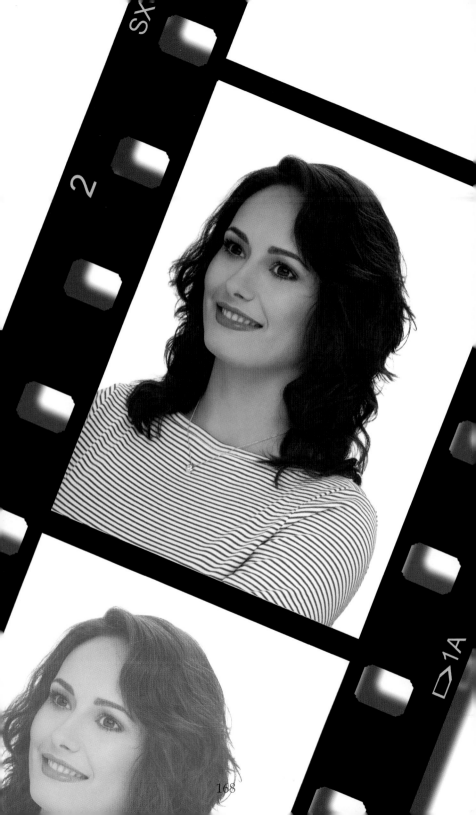

168

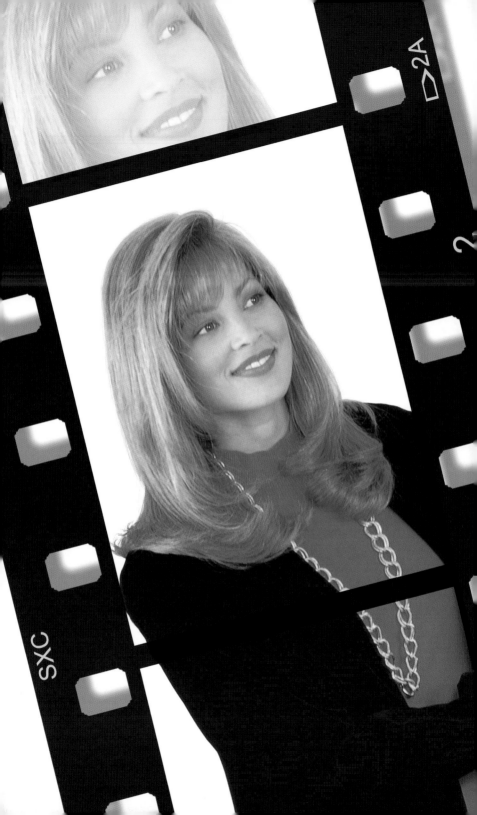

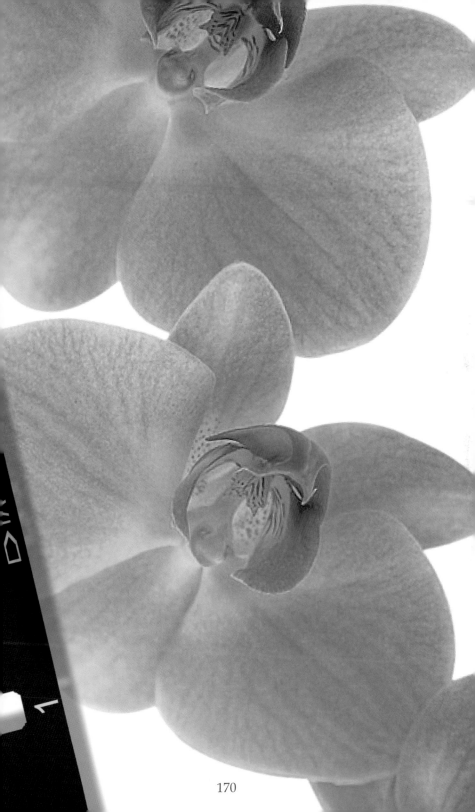

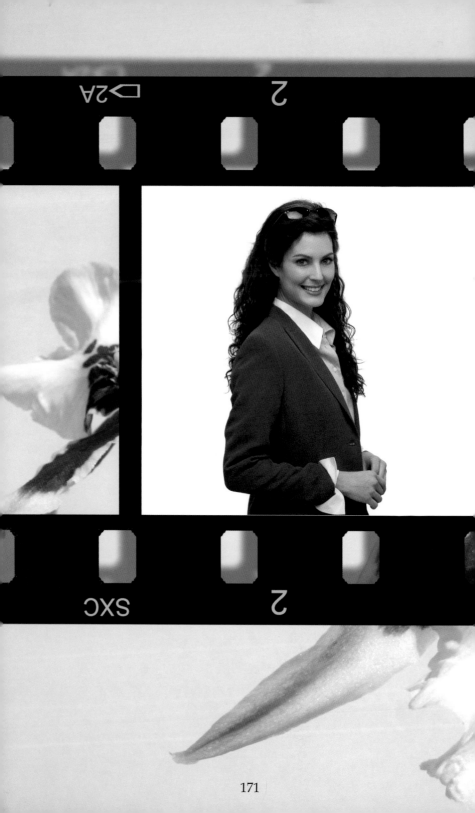

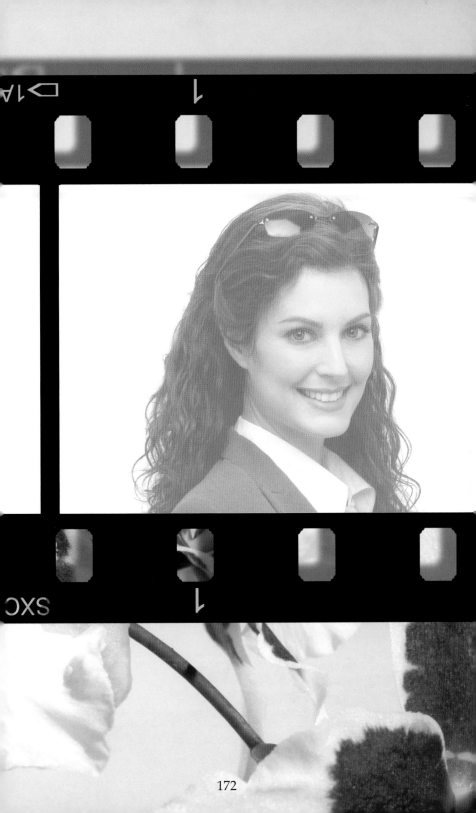

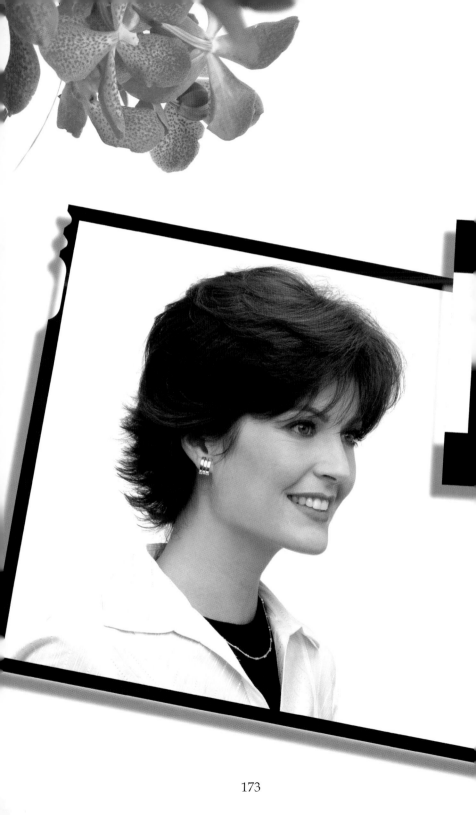

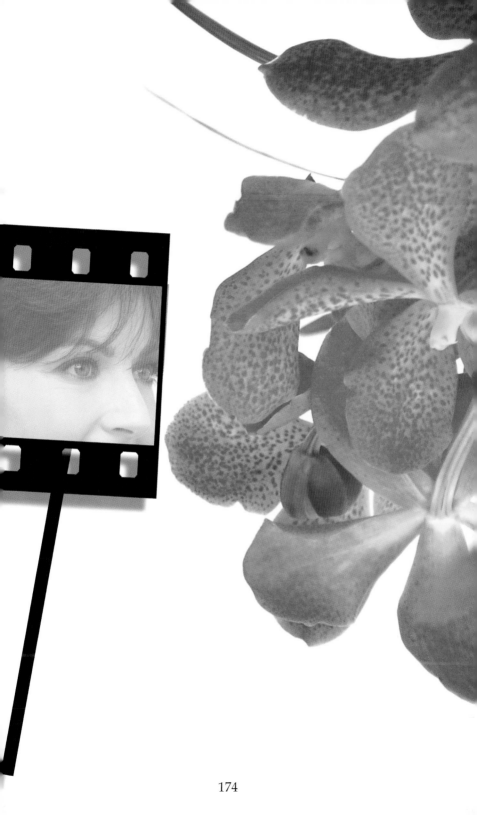

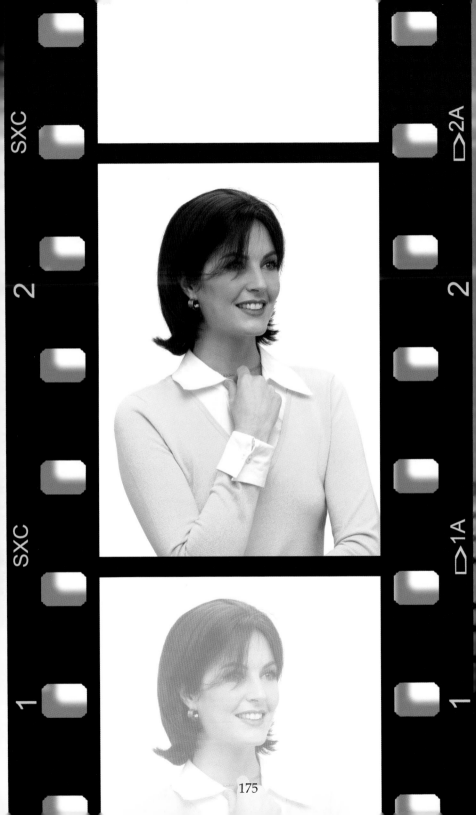

175

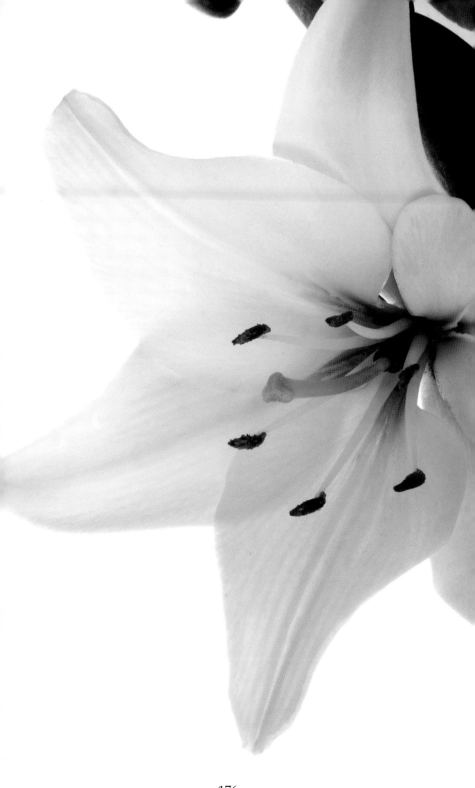

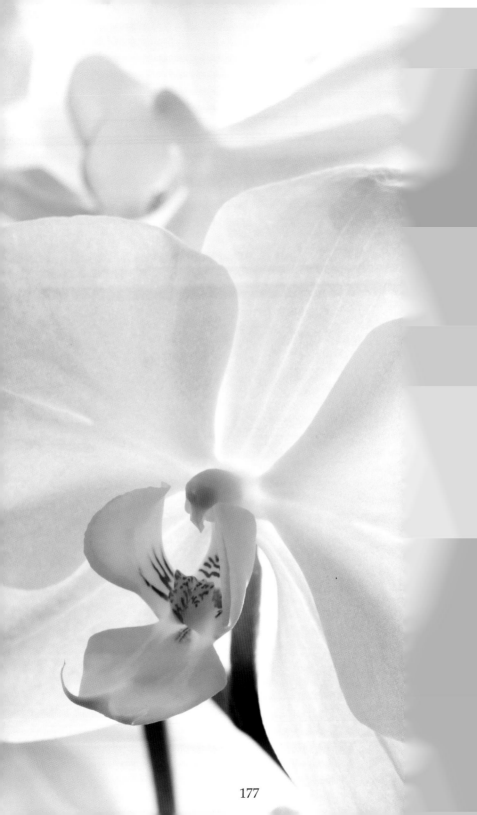

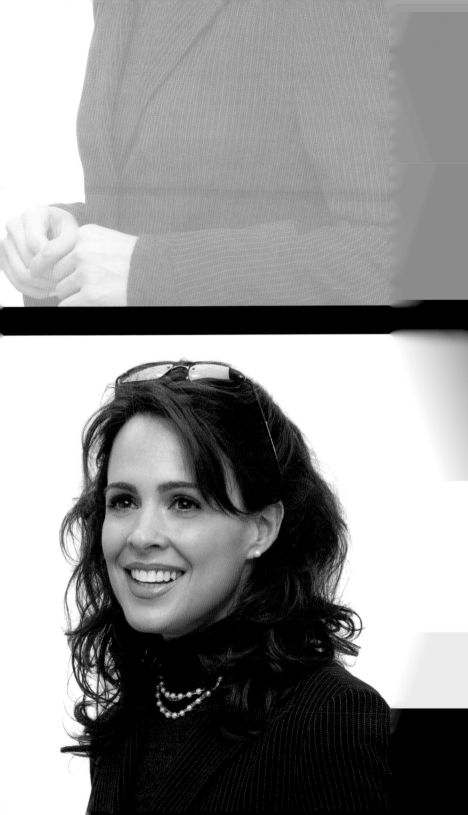

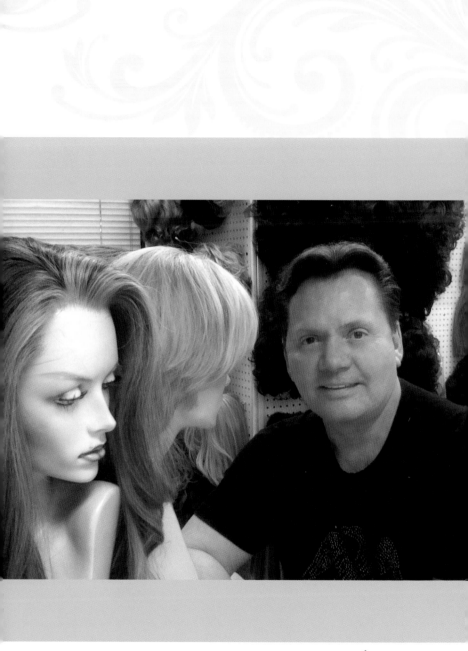

Barry Hendrickson

About the

Author

Barry Hendrickson

Barry's career took off early. He was getting a dollar a cut from his neighborhood clientele in upstate New York at twelve. Fresh out of beauty school, opportunity took him to Las Vegas, where he designed oversized hairpieces for showgirls at Caesar's Palace. He discovered his true calling in the magic of wigs and illusion.

Settling in NYC by 1970, he became equally adept at the fresh and natural as well as his fashion fantasy looks. He created a line of punk hairpieces called Hair Bitz for Jacquelyn International. Cher wore his newly designed black spike wig for her Barbara Walters interview and in many attention getting fitness ads, giving Barry's new punk look instant recognition.

Barry got worldwide media attention on CNN's "Style With Elsa Klencsh" with his "Wig Bar" in the ultra-hip Fiorucci store. His designs were making a bold new fashion statement on record and magazine covers internationally, and on the runways of major designers. The B 52's "Love Shack" video featured his favorite 60's beehives and flips, starting a worldwide trend.

As wig master for the Joffrey Ballet's "Romeo and Juliette", his elaborate creations captured the attention of the entertainment world. Designing for TV and film, Broadway, touring shows, divas and rock bands, it was his dream-come-true to work with many of his favorite stars.

He set up a mini-salon in a chic Upper West Side boutique, with the new name Bitz-n-Pieces. Barry's focus turned to a more natural but equally exciting ready-to-wear concept. He took his "hair as an accessory" concept on the road to stores throughout the country, drawing huge crowds everywhere.

For some, wigs are fun and fashionable. For others, they represent a step towards building a new life. Barry's natural-looking wigs and methods are a welcome solution for clients undergoing chemotherapy.

Recognizing the need for privacy, he opened a beautiful salon on Columbus Avenue in 1991, Barry Hendrickson's Bitz-n-Pieces. American Salon Magazine hailed it as "one of the finest full-service salons in the country". The clientele includes some of the most recognized names in the world.

In a May 1997 article, the New York Times reviewed Barry's unique approach to hair replacement for chemotherapy patients, stating "Hendrickson and company are nothing short of guardian angels." The tremendous response allowed the business to expand to its present location overlooking Columbus Circle.

Continuing to work closely with top manufacturers, Barry foresees ever more lifelike easy-to-wear options for everyday use. These image-enhancing creative illusions will be easy to use. Barry Hendrickson will remain in the forefront of new hair advances.

When clients meet him at the salon, many point to the N.Y.Times article on the wall and echo the now familiar suggestion: "You should write a book." Here it is!

Thanks to...

CONTRIBUTORS:

Jacquelyn International

Follea International

Hair U Wear

Gabor International

Dark Star Lithograph

Global Interprint

PHOTOS ARCHIVES:

Dreamstime.com

Shutterstock.com

Stockxpert.com

Many thanks to Soraya Spahi for her brilliant visualization and designs.

To Joel Clark Kira, for his lighthearted clarification of my words

Special Thanks also to George Mayer, Daniel Hafid, Michael Leigh, Chris Shipman and Ellen Williams for their continued support.

Notes

Notes

Notes

Notes